国务院侨务办公室立项

彭磷基外招生人才培养改革基金资助



# Bilingual Laboratory Manual for Medical Immunology and Microbiology

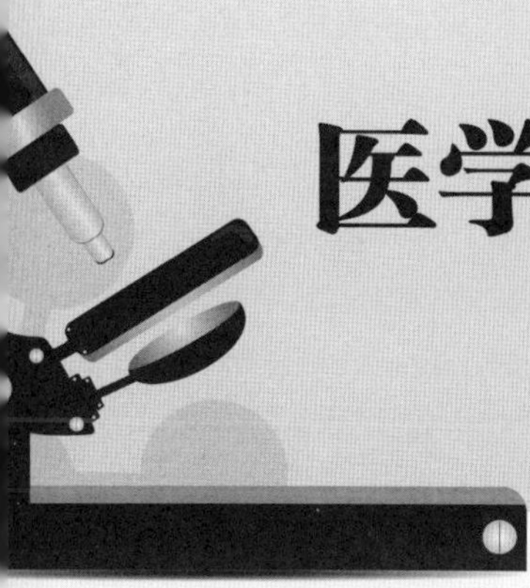

# 医学免疫学与微生物学

## 双语实验指导

江振友　编著

暨南大学出版社
JINAN UNIVERSITY PRESS

中国·广州

**图书在版编目（CIP）数据**

医学免疫学与微生物学双语实验指导 / 江振友编著. —广州：暨南大学出版社，2016.9
ISBN 978-7-5668-1903-1

Ⅰ.①医… Ⅱ.①江… Ⅲ.①医药学—免疫学—实验—双语教学—医学院校—教材 ②医学微生物学—实验—双语教学—医学院校—教材 Ⅳ.①R392-33 ②R37-33

中国版本图书馆 CIP 数据核字（2016）第 183206 号

**医学免疫学与微生物学双语实验指导**
YIXUE MIANYIXUE YU WEISHENGWUXUE SHUANGYU SHIYAN ZHIDAO
**编著者：**江振友

---

**出 版 人：**徐义雄
**责任编辑：**曾鑫华　姚晓莉
**责任校对：**王嘉涵
**责任印制：**汤慧君　王雅琪

**出版发行：**暨南大学出版社（510630）
**电　　话：**总编室（8620） 85221601
营销部（8620） 85225284　85228291　85228292（邮购）
**传　　真：**（8620） 85221583（办公室）　85223774（营销部）
**网　　址：**http: //www.jnupress.com　http: //press.jnu.edu.cn
**排　　版：**广州市天河星辰文化发展部照排中心
**印　　刷：**广东广州日报传媒股份有限公司印务分公司
**开　　本：**787mm × 1092mm　1/16
**印　　张：**12.75
**字　　数：**298 千
**版　　次：**2016 年 9 月第 1 版
**印　　次：**2016 年 9 月第 1 次
**定　　价：**29.80 元

# 前 言

医学是一门实践性很强的学科，而医学实验教学是医学教育的重要组成部分，是保证和提高医学人才培养质量的重要环节和必要手段。随着现代生命科学及各种实验技术的飞速发展，免疫学与微生物学已逐渐渗透到医学各个学科领域，在一些疾病的诊断、治疗和预防上发挥着重要作用，成为推动医学科学乃至整个生命科学向前发展的强大工具。

暨南大学是中国第一所由国家创办的华侨学府，拥有全国最大的国际学院，是目前全国境外生最多的大学。而英语作为一门国际性语言，在教学中的作用尤为重要，像国际学院、华文学院等都采用双语教学，双语教材的编写迫在眉睫。针对新形势下的教学改革，为了适应中国与国际接轨的步伐，满足高等院校普及双语教学的需要，我们编写了本书。我们对医学免疫学与微生物学实验内容进行了重新分类和组合，保留了部分经典的、传统的基础性实验，新增了部分有利于培养学生综合素质及创新能力的实验。本书旨在通过实验来验证和巩固已学的理论知识，通过实验课基本技能训练，培养学生严谨的科学态度和实事求是、独立思考、实践创新的能力，以及分析和解决问题的能力，为进一步学习其他医学专业课程打下良好的基础。

本书可作为医学专业本科生以及研究生的医学免疫学与微生物学实验教材，也可作为医院、卫生防疫部门中从事临床检验、卫生工作的技术人员的参考用书。

本书在编写过程中，得到了许多朋友、同事及学生的帮助和支持。在此谨向他们表示衷心的感谢。特别感谢王鹏程副教授、王辉副教授对英文部分进行了细致的修改及校对；感谢林晨教授、胡萍副教授对实验设计提出了宝贵的指导意见。

由于实验教学仍处于不断探索之中，书中实验的分类和定性只是我们的一家之见，仅供参考。由于作者水平有限，书中难免有错误和不足之处，恳请广大师生和同行专家批评指正。

江振友

2016 年 5 月

# Preface

Medicine is a practical discipline, and laboratory practice is a very important part in medical education to ensure and enhance the quality of medical student training. With the rapid development in modern life science and laboratory techniques, immunology and microbiology have been applied to multiple fields in medicine, and play an important role in diagnosis, treatment and prevention of many diseases, tremendously promoting the development of medical science, even the whole life science.

Jinan University is the first higher educational institute for overseas Chinese founded by government, and has the biggest International School with the largest number of overseas students. As an international language, English plays an important role in teaching. And bilingual teaching is used in International School and College of Chinese Language, so proper bilingual teaching materials are urgently in need. Aiming at the teaching reform under the new situation, and the need to bring China in line with internationl practice, this book is compiled to meet the need in popularizing bilingual teaching in higher educational institutes. We reclassified and recombined the contents of medical immunology and microbiology lab manual keeping some classical and traditional basic experiments and supplementing some experiments which are conducive to cultivate students' comprehensive qualities and innovation abilities. The purposes of this book are to verify and consolidate the students' theoretic knowledge in lectures through experiments, to train students' rigorous scientific attitudes and the abilities of independent and innovative thinking, and the abilities of analyzing and solving problems based on facts, and to lay solid foundation for study on other medical courses.

This book can be used as a laboratory textbook for medical undergraduate and graduate students in medical immunology and microbiology, and can also be used as a reference book for clinical laboratory technicians and health care personnel in hospitals and centers for disease control and prevention as well.

In the process of writing this book, I get lots of help and support from friends, colleagues and students, and I'm writing to extend my sincere gratitude for all of them. Thanks to Dr. Wang Pengcheng and Dr. Wang Hui in terms of the English section improvement, as well as the valuable experimental design suggestion provided by Dr. Lin Chen and Dr. Hu Ping.

Since experimental teaching is still under exploration, and the selection and classification of the contents in this book are from our own point of view, this is for your reference only. Due to our limited ability, errors and shortcomings are unavoidable in the book, and your criticization and correction are greatly appreciated.

Jiang Zhenyou

in May 2016

# 目　录

# CONTENTS

## Part 2 Medical Microbiology Experiment ······ 75

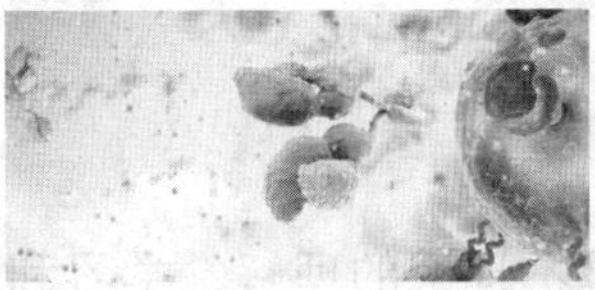

# 第一篇　医学免疫学实验

# Part 1　Medical Immunology Experiment

# 实验须知

## 一、实验课的目的与要求

医学免疫学与微生物学实验课的目的是加强和巩固对课堂基本理论的理解，学习和掌握实验的基本操作技术，提高分析问题和解决问题的能力。为上好实验课，要求同学们做到如下几点：

（1）课前做好充分预习，明确实验的目的、原理、操作方法及注意事项，避免错误的发生。

（2）在实验过程中，严格按照实验步骤和要求进行操作，坚持实验的严肃性、严格性、严谨性。

（3）如实记录实验结果，分析结果，得出结论。对不同的结果要认真分析，找出原因。实验完成后，写好实验报告，及时交给老师批改。

（4）严格遵守实验室规则，防止各种事故的发生。

## 二、实验室规则

实验材料中有些是病原微生物，在实验过程中，必须严肃认真地进行无菌操作，以保证结果准确，并防止实验室感染和环境污染。所以要求同学们认真遵守下列几点：

（1）进入实验室时，先把个人书包放到指定地点，穿好白大衣，实验台上只放实验指导、记录本和文具。非必需的物品请勿带入实验室。

（2）实验室内保持肃静、整洁，不得高声谈笑和随意走动。禁止吸烟、饮食。

（3）实验中如发生割破皮肤或实验材料破损事故，应立即报告教师，进行紧急处理。皮肤破伤可用2%红汞或2%碘酒消毒。如菌液洒到桌面或地面，倾注0.1%新洁尔灭于污染面上，30min后抹去。手上污染活菌，在0.1%新洁尔灭中浸泡10~20min后，再用肥皂水冲洗。

# Instructions

## ⅰ. Purposes and Requirements of the Experiment

The purposes of medical immunology and microbiology experiments are to strengthen and consolidate the understanding of the basic theory of the class, to learn and master the basic operation of experiment technology, to improve the abilities of problem analyzing and solving. In order to have better laboratory courses, students should do all the points as following:

(1) Make full preparation before classes and make clear about the experiment purposes, principles, operation methods and instructions to avoid errors.

(2) In the process of experiment, operate strictly according to the experimental procedures and requirements. Adhere to the seriousness, strictness and rigour of the experiments.

(3) Truthfully record the experimental results. Analyze the results and draw conclusions. Analyze the different results carefully and find out the reasons. After the experiment, write your lab report and hand in it in time to the teacher to correct.

(4) Please obey the rules of the lab strictly in order to prevent all kinds of accidents.

## ⅱ. Rules and Regulations of the Laboratory

Some of the experiment materials are pathogenic microorganisms. To ensure that the results are accurate, and prevent the laboratory infection and environmental pollution, we must be strict with aseptic operation in the process of experiment. So students should carefully obey the following points:

(1) Upon entering the laboratory, put your personal bag into the designated place at first. Then you need to put on a lab coat. Only experiment guidance, notebooks and stationery can be put on the laboratory bench. Don't take non-essential items into the laboratory.

(2) Keep the laboratory quiet and clean. Do not shout or wander. No smoking or eating.

(3) If you cut yourself or break the materials in the experiment, report to the teacher for emergency treatments immediately. Disinfect the broken skin with 2% mercurochrome or 2% iodine. If the bacteria liquid flows on desktop or ground, pour 0.1% bromogeramine on the surface of pollution and wipe it off after 30 minutes. If the living bacterium pollutes your hands, soak them in 0.1% bromogeramine for 10–20 minutes, and then wash with soap water.

(4) The used equipment with bacteria and cultures should be placed in the designated place. Straws which are used to stick bacteria liquid should be put into the barrels with

(4) 用过的有菌器材和培养物放于指定地点，吸过菌液的吸管放在装有消毒液的桶内，载片用后立即放到消毒缸内，不得弃置桌上。接种环使用后应立即于酒精灯火焰上烧灼灭菌。

(5) 爱护实验器材，注意节约实验药品。实验器材如有破损，应立即报告教师，等候处理。易燃物品 (酒精、二甲苯等) 请勿接近火源；酒精灯不可互相直接点燃；如遇火险，先关掉电源，再用湿布或沙土覆盖灭火。

(6) 实验结束后，将实验台整理清洁，再洗手消毒后离去。值日生打扫好室内卫生，关好水电门窗，以防发生安全事故。

disinfection liquid. Put the used slides into disinfection cylinder immediately. Do not put them on the table. Burning the inoculation loops which have been used on the alcohol lamp flame for sterilization immediately.

(5) Take good care of equipment. Don't waste experimental reagents. If there is any damage on the experimental equipment, report to the teacher immediately and wait for instructions. Don't put the flammable items (alcohol, xylene, etc.) close to the fire. Alcohol lamp shall not directly ignite with each other. In case of fire, turn off the power supply first, and then cover wet cloth or sand to put out fire.

(6) After the experiment, clean the laboratory bench, wash and disinfect hands before you leave. The students on duty should do the indoor cleaning. Close the doors and windows, and cut off water and electricity to prevent the occurrence of safety accidents.

# 实验一　凝集反应

颗粒性抗原与相应抗体以合适的比例发生特异性反应时，在一定温度和电解质存在的条件下，形成肉眼可见的凝集物，称为凝集反应（agglutination reaction）。凝集反应主要分为直接凝集反应（direct agglutination reaction）和间接凝集反应（indirect agglutination reaction）两大类（图 1）。

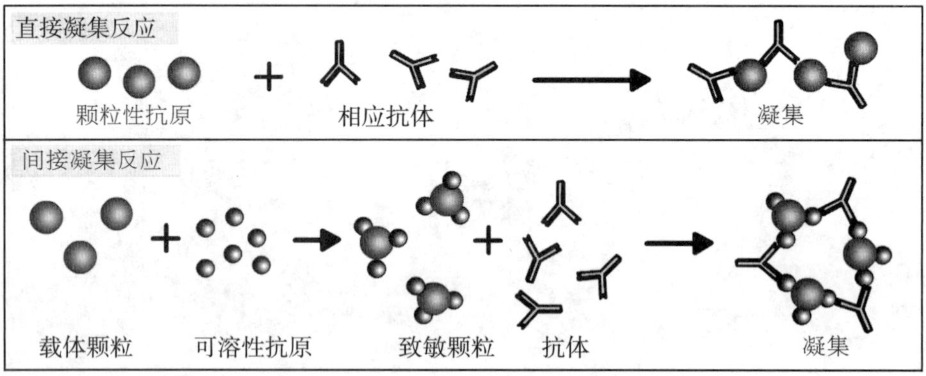


**图 1　凝集反应**

## 一、直接凝集反应

细菌、立克次体、钩端螺旋体和红细胞等颗粒性抗原，在适当电解质参与下可直接与相应抗体结合出现凝集，称为直接凝集反应。凝集反应中的抗原称为凝集原，抗体称为凝集素。常用的凝集实验有玻片法和试管法两种。

ABO 血型测定（玻片凝集反应）

**【实验目的】**

掌握玻片凝集反应的原理、方法、结果判定及应用。

# Ⅰ. Agglutination Reaction

Under the conditions of proper temperature and electrolytes, antigens in particulate form react with the corresponding antibodies to form visible clumps. This process is called an agglutination reaction. Agglutination reaction is mainly divided into two categories: direct agglutination reaction and indirect agglutination reaction (Figure 1).

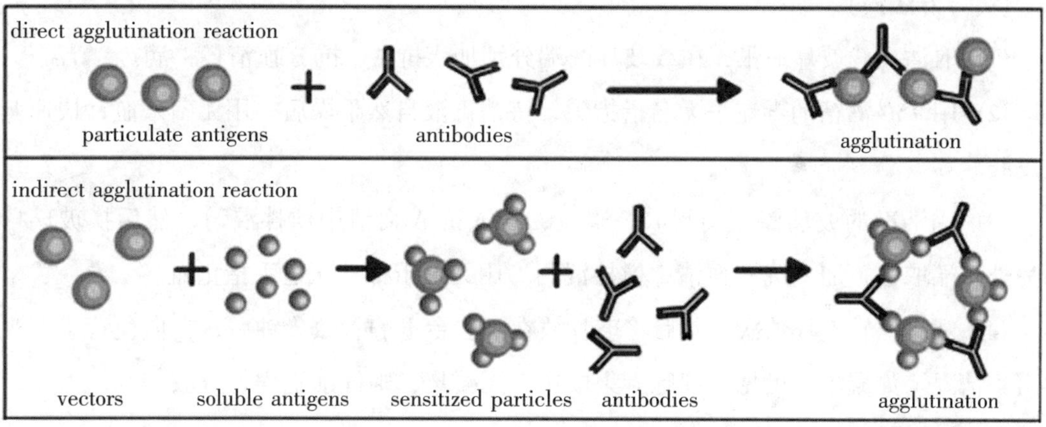


Figure 1 Agglutination Reaction

## ⅰ. Direct Agglutination Reaction

Under the participation of proper electrolytes, bacteria, rickettsia, leptospira, red blood cells and other particulate antigens can directly react with the corresponding antibodies with the appearance of agglutination. This process is called direct agglutination reaction. In the process of agglutination reaction, the antigen is called agglutinogen, and antibody is called agglutinin. Commonly, slide method and tube method are two approaches to the agglutination test.

### ABO Blood Group Determination (Slide Agglutination Reaction)

**【Aim】**

To master the principle, method, result determination and application of slide agglutination reaction.

**【实验原理】**

ABO血型系统是按照血液中红细胞表面的抗原分子来命名的。人类ABO血型抗原有两种：A抗原和B抗原。A型血红细胞表面有A抗原，B型血红细胞表面有B抗原，AB型血红细胞表面有A、B两种抗原，O型血红细胞表面既无A抗原也无B抗原。ABO血型测定根据人类红细胞表面有不同的血型抗原，用已知的抗A和抗B单克隆抗体，与受试者红细胞上的相应抗原直接做玻片凝集实验，根据红细胞是否出现凝集，可判定受试者的血型。

**【实验器材】**

(1) 标准抗A和抗B血清（抗A为蓝色，抗B为黄色）、生理盐水（NS)、碘酒、75%酒精。

(2) 洁净载玻片、试管、无菌采血针、消毒棉签等。

**【实验方法】**

(1) 取洁净载玻片一张，在载玻片两端分别加入抗A、抗B血清各一滴。

(2) 用75%酒精消毒左手无名指指尖，待消毒液自然干燥后，用无菌采血针快速刺破皮肤。

(3) 用洁净的玻璃棒一端刮取一滴血，加入抗A血清中搅拌混匀，然后换玻璃棒的另外一端取血，加入抗B血清中搅拌混匀。用无菌干棉签压迫手指止血。

(4) 观察摇转玻片数次，然后将玻片放在实验台上静置数分钟后，在白色背景下观察凝集情况。如凝集，可见红细胞凝集成块；无凝集，则红细胞均匀分散。

**【实验结果】**

红细胞凝集成块，周围液体澄清者为阳性（+)；红细胞仍均匀分散、无凝集者为阴性（–)。与抗A血清发生凝集者为A型血；与抗B血清发生凝集者为B型血；与抗A、抗B血清均发生凝集者为AB型血；与抗A、抗B血清均不发生凝集者为O型血。

**【注意事项】**

(1) 载玻片上划分A、B两区，切忌让两种诊断血清混合；牙签的两端不可混用。待测血样与诊断血清调匀后，不要再用牙签搅动，以免影响大凝集块形成。

(2) 用采血针刺手指时，应捏紧被刺部位，动作要迅速，刺入深度要适宜；用手指挤血时，应从刺入点稍远端向近端挤压。

(3) 血滴要迅速加入诊断血清并混匀，以防血液自然凝固。

**【Principle】**

The ABO blood grouping system is based on antigen molecules present on the surface of RBC (red blood cells). There are two types of human ABO blood group antigens: A-antigen and B-antigen. Type A red blood cells have A-antigen on cell surface, and type B red blood cells have B-antigen on cell surface. There are both A-antigen and B-antigen presenting on type AB red blood cells, while neither A-antigen nor B-antigen is on type O red blood cell surface. ABO blood group determination is based on the different antigens on the surface of human red blood cells, therefore, we use known anti-A and anti-B monoclonal antibodies to mix with the antigens of RBC samples to make a direct slide agglutination test. According to whether RBC agglutination appears, we can determine the blood group of the subject.

**【Materials and Equipment】**

(1) Standard anti-A (blue) and anti-B (yellow) blood grouping serums, normal saline (NS), iodine, 75% alcohol.

(2) Clean slides, tubes, sterile lancets, sterilized cotton swab, etc.

**【Procedures】**

(1) Take a clean slide, and add a drop of anti-A and anti-B blood grouping serums on each side of the slide respectively.

(2) Sanitize left ring finger with 75% alcohol, fast puncture the skin with a sterile lancet when the finger is dry.

(3) Collect some blood with a glass rod and transfer blood to both ends of the slide, mix well with antibodies respectively. Stress the finger with a dry sterilized cotton swab to stop bleeding.

(4) Shake the slide several times, and place the slide on the laboratory bench for a few minutes to observe the agglutination on a white background. If agglutination appears, red blood cells will be visibly agglutinated. Otherwise, red blood cells are uniformly dispersed.

**【Results】**

The one red blood cells agglutinated with clear surrounding liquid is positive (+); and the one red blood cells distributed homogeneously with no agglutination is negative (−). Those agglutinated with anti-A blood grouping serum are type A blood; those agglutinated with anti-B blood grouping serum are type B blood; those agglutinated with both anti-A and anti-B blood grouping serums are type AB blood; and those agglutinated with neither anti-A blood grouping serum nor anti-B blood grouping serum are type O blood.

**【Attentions】**

(1) Divide the slide into A and B regions, and the two diagnostic serums are not allowed to be mixed; both ends of the toothpick can not be used together. When the blood samples and diagnostic serums are mixed thoroughly, do not stir with a toothpick, in order not to affect the fomation of large agglutination.

(2) When stinging fingers, you should pinch the stabbed part tightly and act quickly. The blood should be squeezed slightly far from the stabbed point to near the stabbed point.

(3) The blood should be quickly added into diagnostic serums and mixed evenly to

## 二、间接凝集反应

将可溶性抗原或抗体吸附于与免疫无关的载体表面，然后与相应的抗体或抗原反应，形成肉眼可见的凝集物，称为间接凝集反应。其中将抗体吸附于载体表面检测抗原的间接凝集反应，称为反向间接凝集实验。常用作载体的物质有人和多种动物红细胞、聚苯乙烯胶乳颗粒、活性炭粒、金黄色葡萄球菌 A 蛋白（SPA）等。

### 甲苯胺红不加热血清实验

**【实验目的】**

熟悉正向间接凝集实验的原理，了解其临床应用。

**【实验原理】**

用可溶性抗原致敏载体检测相应抗体。常用的载体有人 O 型红细胞、绵羊红细胞、细菌、胶乳颗粒、活性炭及甲苯胺红颗粒等。本实验以检测梅毒反应素为例介绍甲苯胺红不加热血清实验（toluidine red unheated serum test, TRUST），该实验是以甲苯胺红颗粒为载体的间接凝集反应。受梅毒螺旋体感染后，机体可产生一种非特异性抗体——反应素，该抗体能与牛心肌磷脂抗原发生交叉反应。将处理后的可溶性牛心肌磷脂抗原吸附到甲苯胺红载体颗粒表面致敏以检测反应素，常用于梅毒的初筛。

**【实验器材】**

（1）TRUST 试剂。

（2）待测血清，阳性对照血清、阴性对照血清。

（3）TRUST 实验专用卡片。

（4）9 号无斜面针头（滴加 TRUST 试剂用）。

**【实验方法】**

1.定性实验

（1）分别吸取 50μL 梅毒阳性对照血清和阴性对照血清，均匀铺加在纸卡的两个圆圈中。

（2）取待检血清或血浆 50μL（不需灭活）置于纸卡的另一个圆圈中。

（3）用专用滴管及针头分别垂直滴加 TRUST 试剂 1 滴于上述血清中。

（4）按每分钟 100 转摇动 8 分钟，肉眼观察结果。

2.定量实验

将待检血清用生理盐水做倍比稀释，然后按上述定性方法进行实验，以呈现明显凝集反应的最高稀释度作为该血清的凝集效价。

prevent blood coagulation.

## ii. Indirect Agglutination Reaction

Soluble antigen or antibody adsorbed on the surface of an irrelevant immune carrier reacts with the corresponding antibody or antigen to form visible agglutination. This is called indirect agglutination reaction. The indirect agglutination reaction with antibody adsorbed on the surface of carriers is called reverse indirect agglutination test. Commonly used carriers include human and animal red blood cells, polystyrene latex particles, activated carbon particles, and *Staphylococcus aureus* protein A (SPA), etc.

### Toluidine Red Unheated Serum Test (TRUST)

**【Aim】**

To get familiar with experiment principle of positive indirect agglutination test, and understand its clinical application.

**【Principle】**

It's an experiment using soluble antigen absorbed on carriers to detect the corresponding antibodies. Common carriers include human type O red blood cells, sheep red blood cells, bacteria, latex particles, activated carbon and toluidine red particles, etc. The toluidine red unheated serum test (TRUST) is an indirect agglutination reaction, using toluidine red particles as the carrier to detect reagin in syphilis. Treponema pallidum infection can elicit non-specific antibodies. The antibodies, called reagin, can cross react with phospholipid antigen extracted from bovine heart muscle. The processed soluble bovine phospholipid antigen is absorbed on the surface of toluidine red carrier particles to detect reagin, and TRUST is commonly used in the screening of syphilis.

**【Materials and Equipment】**

(1) TRUST reagent.

(2) Testing serums, positive and negative control serums.

(3) Special card for TRUST test.

(4) NO. 9 unbeveled needle (to drop the TRUST reagent).

**【Procedures】**

#### 1. Qualitative test

(1) Drop 50 microliters of syphilis positive and negative control serums evenly in circles of testing cards, respectively.

(2) Take 50 microliters of testing serums or plasma (no need to be inactivated) and place in another circle.

(3) Vertically add 1 drop of TRUST reagent into the control serums and testing serums.

(4) Shake for 8 minutes at the speed of 100 RPM (revolutions per minute), and observe results.

#### 2. Quantitative test

The testing serums are diluted with normal saline, then perform test according to the

**【实验结果】**

(1) 阳性反应可见中等或大的红色凝集块。

(2) 弱阳性反应可见散在的细小红色凝集块。

(3) 阴性反应无颗粒凝集，液体浑浊，或仅见粗糙的红色颗粒集聚中央。

above qualitative method. The highest dilution of which obvious agglutination reaction shows is used as agglutination titer of serums.

**【Results】**

(1) Positive reaction shows visible medium or large red clots.

(2) Small red clots can be seen scattered in the weak positive reaction.

(3) Negative reaction has no particle agglutination, the fluid is turbid, or only has rough red particles gathering in the center.

# 实验二 沉淀反应

可溶性抗原与相应抗体以合适的比例发生特异性反应时，在一定温度和电解质存在的条件下，形成肉眼可见的沉淀物，称为沉淀反应。沉淀反应的抗原可以是多糖、蛋白质、脂类等。

## 一、单向免疫琼脂扩散实验

**【实验目的】**

掌握单向免疫琼脂扩散实验的原理及应用，熟悉其基本操作方法。

**【实验原理】**

通常是用已知抗体测定未知抗原。将一定量的抗体混合于琼脂内，倾注于玻片上，凝固后打孔，并在孔中加入定量的抗原，由于琼脂中抗体浓度分布均匀，故只有孔中抗原向四周扩散，与琼脂中相应抗体相遇并结合，在比例合适处形成白色沉淀环。沉淀环的直径大小与抗原的浓度成正比。以不同浓度的标准抗原与固定浓度的抗血清反应，将测得的沉淀环直径作为纵坐标，以抗原浓度为横坐标，绘制标准曲线，量取待检抗原的沉淀环直径，即可从标准曲线中求得其含量（图 2）。该实验主要用于检测标本中的各种 Ig 含量、血清中的补体成分和甲胎蛋白的含量。

# Ⅱ. Precipitation Reaction

Precipitation reaction occurs when soluble antigen combines with corresponding antibody in the appropriate proportion with the presence of electrolytes, which produces visible precipitates at a certain temperature. Antigens in the precipitation reaction include polysaccharide, protein and lipid, etc.

## ⅰ. Single Agar Immunodiffusion Test

**【Aim】**

To master the principle of single agar immunodiffusion test and its application, be familiar with its basic methods of operation.

**【Principle】**

Usually it is used to measure unknown antigen by known antibody. Mix certain quantity of antibody with agar and pour on slide to make an agar plate containing antibody. Cut wells after agar concretion. Then add unknown antigen into wells. Since antibody concentration is evenly distributed, and antigen diffuses outward from wells and meets corresponding antibody in the agar, a white precipitation circle is formed at the place where antigen and antibody are of appropriate proportion. The diameter of precipitation circle shows a linear relationship with the concentration of antigen. The standard curve can be obtained by using the diameter of the precipitation circle as ordinate and the concentration of standard antigen as abscissa. If we measure the diameter of the precipitation circle of the unknown antigen, we can tell its concentration from the standard curve (Figure 2). This test is mainly used to measure the content of a variety kinds of Ig, complement and AFP in serum.

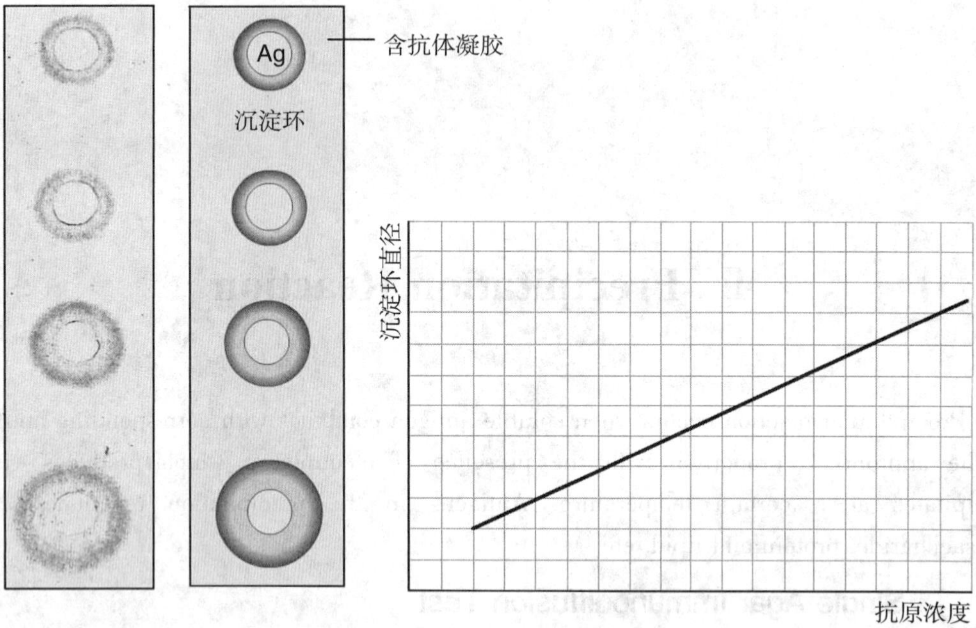


**图 2　单向免疫琼脂扩散实验**

**【实验器材】**

(1) 2%离子琼脂或生理盐水琼脂（含 2%$NaN_3$）、标准马抗人 IgG 血清（抗体）、工作标准参考蛋白、pH7.2 PBS。

(2) 打孔器（孔径 3mm）及打孔模板、微量加样器及塑料吸头、尖吸管及橡皮吸头、载玻片、湿盒（附湿纱布或泡沫塑料）。

(3) 已制备好的含有 1%马抗人 IgG 抗体的琼脂板、1:50 稀释的待检血清标本。

**【实验方法】**

(1) 把马抗人 IgG 血清按一定比例（预试测定好的）混合在融化的琼脂中（水浴 56~60℃），在玻片上浇注成 2mm 厚的琼脂板。

(2) 琼脂冷凝后隔一定距离（约 1.5cm）在琼脂板上打孔。

(3) 用微量加样器从最低浓度开始把四个已知浓度的标准马抗人 IgG 溶液自右向左分别加到相应的几个孔中，每孔 10μL，余孔加入待检血清标本。

(4) 待抗原溶液完全被吸收到琼脂层中，把琼脂板放入湿盒中，然后置于 37℃温箱内，24h 后观察结果。

**【实验结果】**

(1) 取出琼脂板，即可见清晰的乳白色沉淀环。测沉淀环直径并记录。

(2) 用已知抗原浓度为横坐标，沉淀环直径为纵坐标，在半对数纸上作图，绘制标

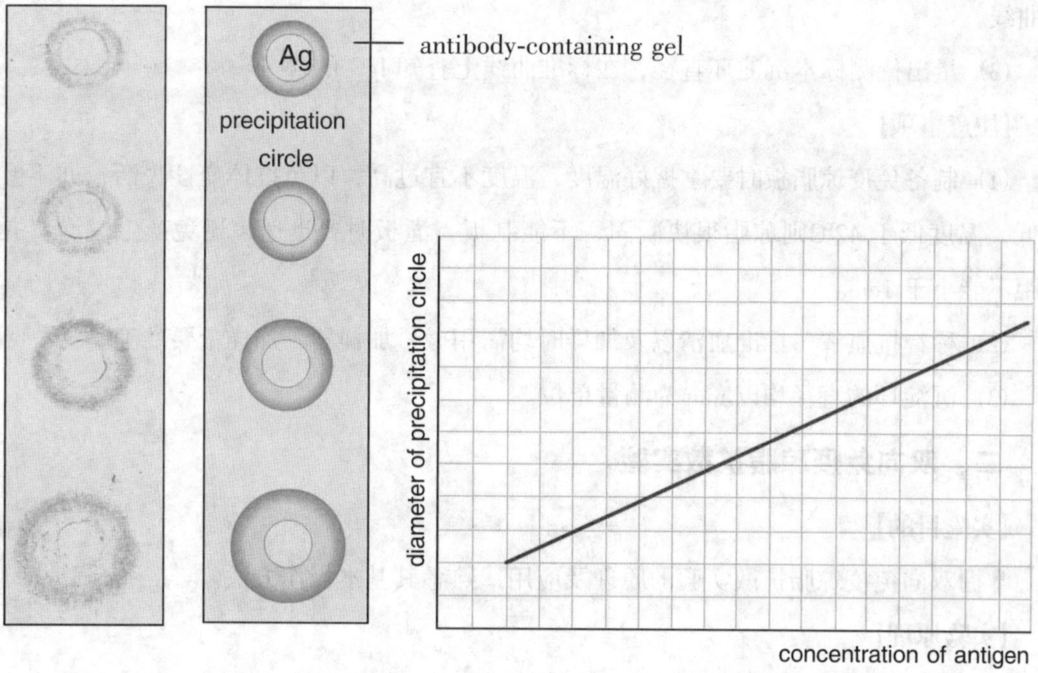


Figure 2 Single Agar Immunodiffusion Test

【Materials and Equipment】

(1) 2% ionic agar or normal saline agar (contains 2%$NaN_3$), standard anti-human IgG serum (antibody) produced in horse, standard reference protein, pH7.2 PBS.

(2) Puncher(well diameter=3mm) and template, micropipettes and plastic tips, pipettes and rubber tips, slides, moist chamber (include wet gauze or polyfoam).

(3) The agar slides mixed with 1% anti-human IgG antibody produced in horse, 1:50 dilution of the testing serum.

【Procedures】

(1) Mix anti-human IgG serum produced in horse properly with melted agar at 56–60℃. Then pour solution on slide immediately to make a 2mm thick layer of agar.

(2) Cut wells with the puncher in the agar slide after agar concretion. The distance among wells is about 1.5cm.

(3) Respectively from the lowest concentration add the four known concentration of standard anti-human IgG solution by micropipettes into agar wells from right to left. Respectively add 10μL of testing serum into the rest wells.

(4) Place the agar slide in a moist chamber, then put the moist chamber in 37℃ thermostat for 24h after the antigen solution is completely absorbed into the agar layer.

【Results】

(1) Take out the agar slide, you will find milky white precipitation circle. Measure the diameter and write it down.

(2) Draw a standard curve by using the concentration of antigen as abscissa and the

准曲线。

(3) 量出待测标本沉淀环直径，在标准曲线上查知 IgG 的含量。

**【注意事项】**

(1) 制备免疫琼脂板时要掌握好温度，温度不宜过高，以免抗体变性失活；亦不宜太低，温度低于 42℃则琼脂很快凝固，不能制板。灌板时要迅速，避免产生气泡。孔间距不能小于 1cm。

(2) 稀释抗血清、标准血清以及加样时均需用微量加样器，加样量要准确。

(3) 沉淀环的直径均以 mm 为测量单位。

## 二、双向免疫琼脂扩散实验

**【实验目的】**

掌握双向免疫琼脂扩散实验的原理及应用，熟悉其基本操作方法。

**【实验原理】**

双向免疫琼脂扩散（double agar immunodiffusion）是指可溶性抗原与相应抗体在半固体琼脂介质中相互扩散，彼此相遇后形成一定类型的特异性沉淀线。沉淀线的特征与位置取决于抗原与抗体的特异性、相互间比例，以及分子大小和扩散速度。依据沉淀线的形态、清晰度及位置可了解抗原或抗体的若干性质，如浓度、特异性等。此实验可检测抗原或抗体的纯度，滴定抗体的效价，也可用已知抗原（抗体）检测和分析未知抗体（抗原）（图 3）。临床上常用于检测甲胎蛋白（AFP），其结果可作为原发性肝癌的重要诊断指标。

diameter of the precipitation circle as ordinate on the semi-logarithmic paper.

(3) Measure the diameter of the precipitation circle of the testing sample and the concentration of IgG can be calculated from the standard curve.

**【Attentions】**

(1) When preparing the agar slide, you must keep a proper temperature. The temperature of the agar solution shouldn't be too high in order to avoid denaturalization and inactivation of the antibody. And it shouldn't be too low in order to avoid the agar solidification before spreading out on the slide because the agar will solidify soon if the temperature is below 42℃. The agar must be added rapidly to avoid the bubble formation. The distance between adjacent wells should be beyond 1cm.

(2) When diluting antiserum and standard serum or adding the samples, micropipettes must be used. The samples must be added accurately.

(3) The diameter of the precipitation circle is measured in mm.

## ii. Double Agar Immunodiffusion Test

**【Aim】**

To master the principle of double agar immunodiffusion test and its application, be familiar with its basic methods of operation.

**【Principle】**

Double agar immunodiffusion is a test in which both soluble antigen and corresponding antibody diffuse in the semisolid agar. So visible precipitation line appears where antigen and antibody are of appropriate proportion. The characteristics and location of the precipitation line can be analyzed according to antigen and antibody's specificity, proportion as well as their molecular size and diffusion velocity. On the basis of precipitation line's shape, clarity and location, we can understand several properties of antigen or antibody, such as concentration, specificity, etc. The test can determine the purity of antigen and antibody, measure the titer of antibody, and can use a known antigen (antibody) to detect and analyze an unknown antibody (antigen)(Figure 3). It is often clinically used to detect α-fetoprotein (AFP), and the result can be used as an important diagnostic index of primary liver cancer.

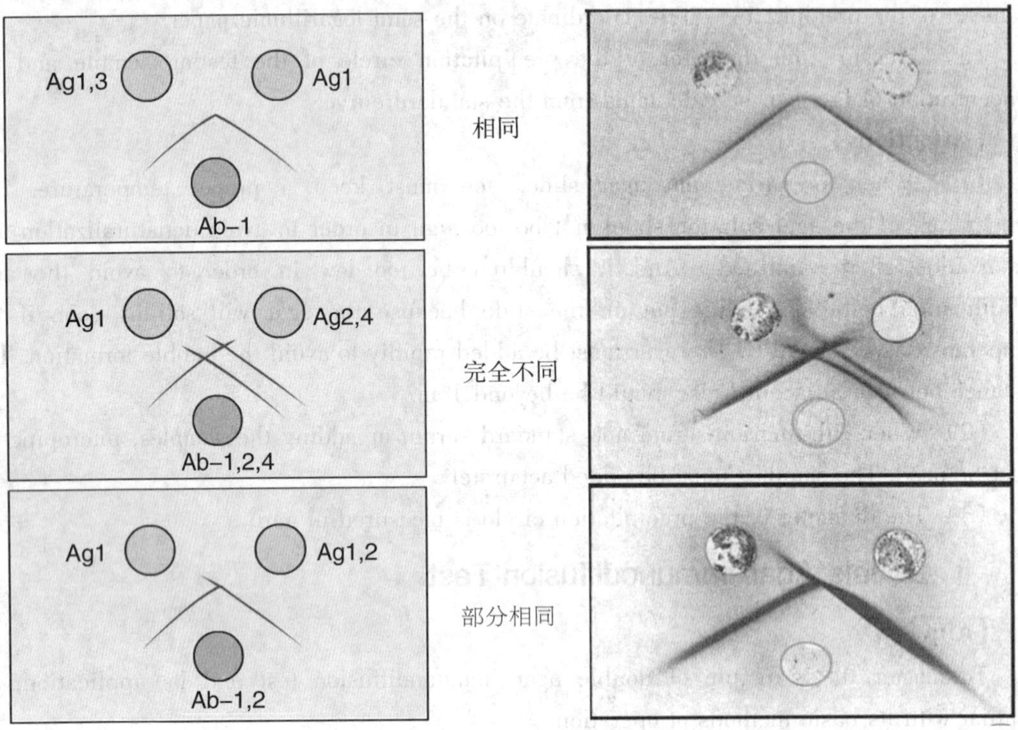


**图 3 双向免疫琼脂扩散实验**

**【实验器材】**

(1) 1%生理盐水琼脂管（每管 4~5mL）、抗 HBsAg 抗体（诊断血清）、HBsAg 阳性血清、待检血清甲、待检血清乙、HBsAg 阴性血清、生理盐水。

(2) 载玻片、打孔器及打孔模板、微量加样器及塑料吸头、湿盒、温箱。

**【实验方法】**

(1) 融化 1%生理盐水琼脂。

(2) 将载玻片置于水平桌面上，倾注已融化琼脂约 4mL，将其制成厚度约为 1.5mm 的琼脂板。注意：倾注速度不要过快，以免琼脂溢出载玻片；倾注过程务必连续，以保证琼脂板均匀、平滑。

(3) 琼脂凝固后，将梅花形打孔模板置于琼脂板下，然后用打孔器打孔。

(4) 用微量加样器分别加各样品材料 10μL 于各孔中。注意每加一样品均需更换吸头，以防止交叉污染，影响实验结果。

(5) 做好标记，放入湿盒中，然后置于 37℃温箱内，24h 后观察结果。

**【实验结果】**

阳性待检血清、阳性对照血清与抗体之间形成融合性沉淀线，说明两孔中抗原相

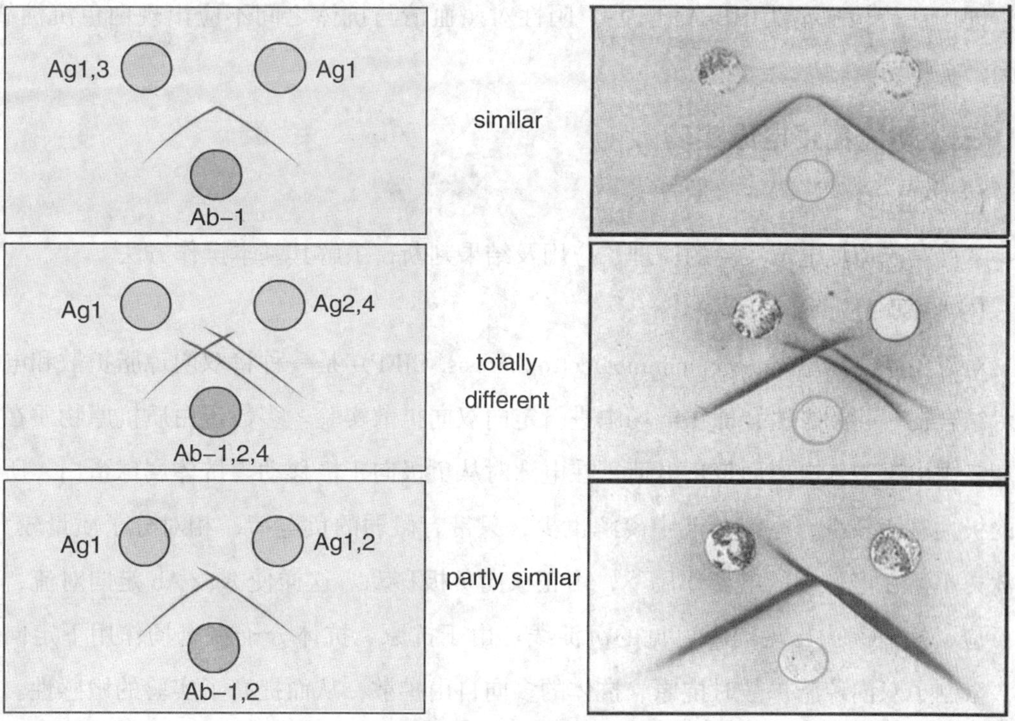


Figure 3 Double Agar Immunodiffusion Test

【Materials and Equipment】

(1) 1% normal saline agar's tubes (4–5mL per tube), Anti-HBsAg antibody (diagnostic serum), HBsAg positive serum, testing serum 1 and serum 2, HBsAg negative serum, normal saline.

(2) Slides, puncher and template, micropipettes and plastic tips, moist chamber, thermostat.

【Procedures】

(1) Melt 1% normal saline agar.

(2) Put the slide on the horizontal table, and about 4mL of melted agar is poured on the slide, the thickness of agar is about 1.5mm. Pay attention to the speed of pouring, if the speed is too fast, the agar may overflow from the slide. And the process must be continuous to ensure that the agar slide is even.

(3) Put the template under agar slide, and punch wells in the solidified agar. The pattern of wells looks like a plum blossom.

(4) Add each of samples respectively into corresponding well by micropipettes, 10μL per well. Change tips to avoid cross-contamination which will affect the result of the test.

(5) Label the samples, and put them into moist chamber and then put the moist chamber in 37℃ thermostat for 24h. Then observe the results.

【Results】

If the positive testing serum or positive control serum produces a precipitation line with

同，即阳性待检血清为 HBsAg 阳性。阴性对照血清与抗体之间不应出现白色沉淀线，否则，实验无效。

## 三、对流免疫电泳实验

【实验目的】

掌握对流免疫电泳实验的原理、应用及结果判断，了解其基本操作方法。

【实验原理】

对流免疫电泳（counter immunoelectrophoresis, CIEP）是一种将双向琼脂扩散和电泳技术结合在一起的方法，即在电场中进行定向双向扩散实验。多数蛋白质抗原物质在碱性环境中由于羧基电离而带负电荷，在电泳时从负极向正极移动。抗体属球蛋白，所暴露的极性基团较少，在缓冲液中离解也少，只带有微弱的负电荷，相对分子质量较大，电泳力小，在电场中的电渗作用下，由正极向负极移动。这样使 Ag/Ab 定向对流，发生反应，短时间内出现肉眼可见的沉淀线。由于抗原、抗体分子在电场作用下定向运动，限制了双向琼脂扩散时抗原、抗体的多向自由扩散，从而提高了实验的敏感性。根据沉淀线的数量、位置，分析标本中所含抗原的性质（图 4）。

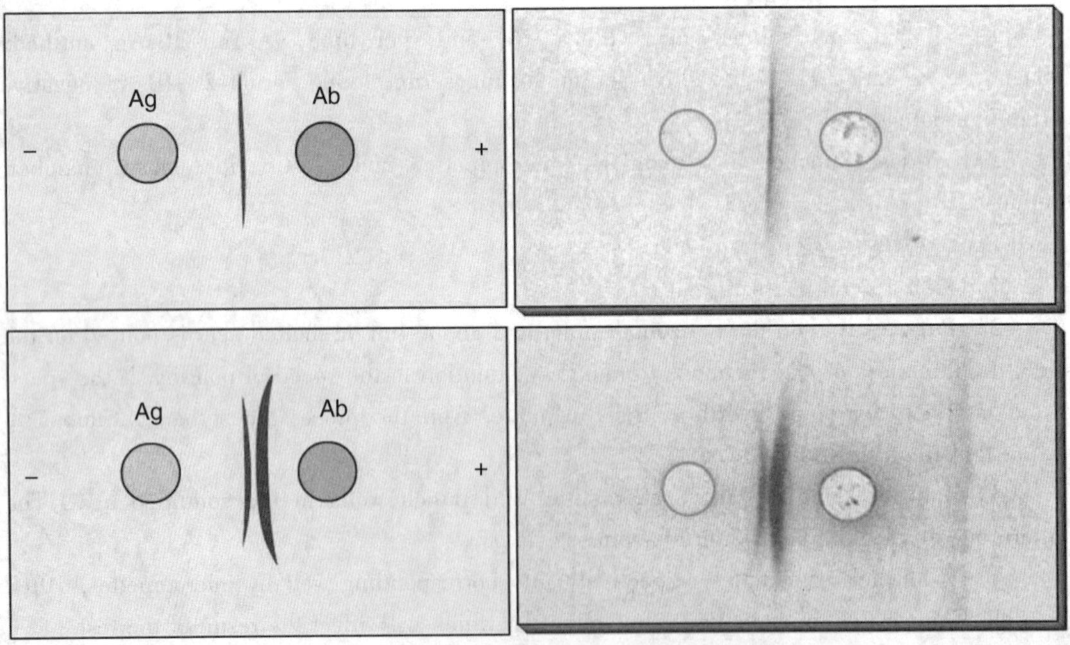


图 4 对流免疫电泳实验

the corresponding antibody, it indicates that the antigens in the two wells are identical, and testing serum is HBsAg positive. Negative control serum doesn't produce a white precipitation line with corresponding antibody, otherwise, this test fails.

## iii. Counter Immunoelectrophoresis Test

**【Aim】**

To master the principle of counter immunoelectrophoresis test and its application and result detection, be familiar with its basic methods of operation.

**【Principle】**

Counter immunoelectrophoresis is a method that combines the double agar diffusion with electrophoresis. The double diffusion experiment is carried out in the electric field. Most of the protein antigens in alkaline environment are negatively charged due to ionization of the carboxyl. It can move from cathode to anode during the electrophoresis. Antibody is globulin, with fewer exposed polar groups and less dissociation in buffer, which makes it only weakly negatively-charged. Antibody has higher molecular weight, but electrophoretic force is lower. Because of electroosmosis in the electric field, it will move from anode to cathode. So Ag/Ab directional convection occurs. Ag reacts with Ab, in which visible precipitation lines appear in a short time. Because the antigen and antibody molecules produce oriented movement in the electric field, which limits free multi-directional diffusion of antigen in double agar diffusion so as to improve the sensitivity of the test. According to the amount and the location of precipitation lines, the property of antigen of the samples can be analyzed (Figure 4).

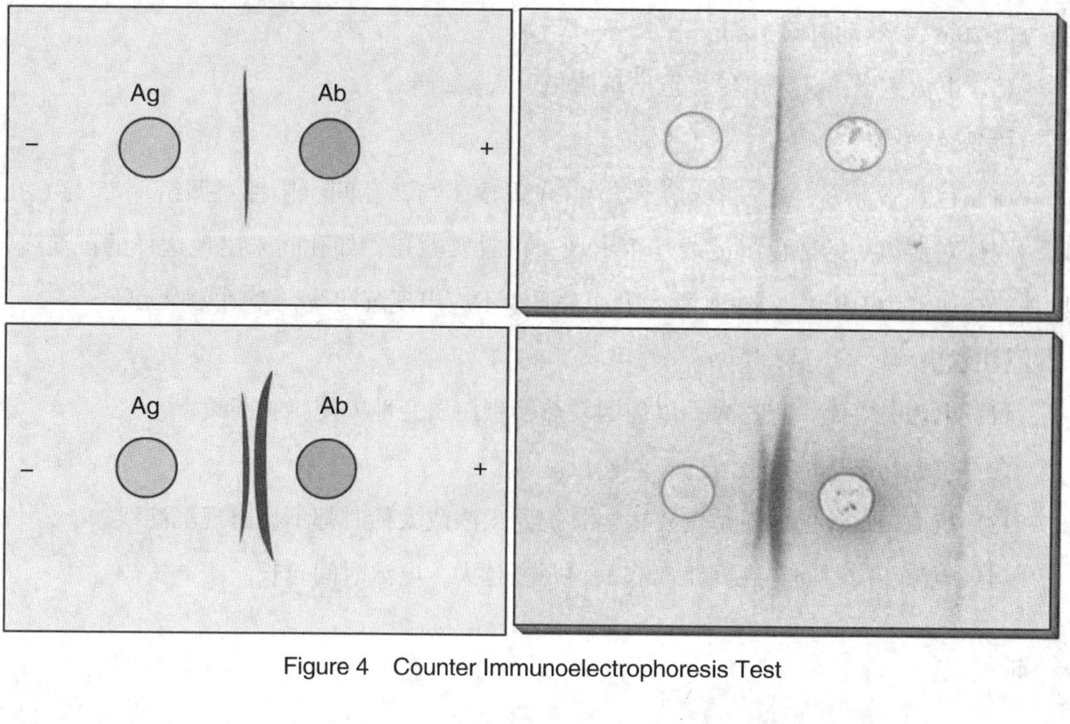


Figure 4 Counter Immunoelectrophoresis Test

**【实验器材】**

(1) 1%离子琼脂（在 pH8.6 巴比妥缓冲液中加入等量蒸馏水，再加入 1%琼脂。溶解后用脱脂棉过滤、分装，实验前加热溶解备用）。

(2) 抗 HBsAg 抗体（诊断血清）、HBsAg 阳性血清、待检血清、HBsAg 阴性血清、生理盐水。

(3) 微量加样器及塑料吸头、尖吸管及橡皮吸头、载玻片、打孔器及打孔模板。

(4) 电泳槽、电泳仪（将 pH8.6 巴比妥缓冲液注入电泳槽内，并将滤纸裁至适当长度和宽度以备搭桥使用）。

**【实验方法】**

(1) 将融化的 1%离子琼脂 4~5mL 倾注于玻片上制成琼脂板。

(2) 待琼脂板冷却凝固后，按照打孔模板用打孔器打孔，并用微量加样器加样，各孔中加入各样本 10μL。从上至下分别向左列 2、4、6 孔内加抗 HBsAg 抗体；向右列 3 孔内加待检患者血清，1 孔内加 HBsAg 阳性血清作为阳性对照，5 孔内加 HBsAg 阴性血清作为阴性对照。

(3) 将琼脂板置于电泳槽内，抗原端放阴极侧，抗体端放阳极侧，并将已浸透缓冲液的滤纸一端覆盖于琼脂板两侧各约 0.5cm，另一端浸于电泳液中。

(4) 接通电源，电压、电流及电泳时间视仪器性能而定。一般地，电压 6V/cm，电流每板 20mA，泳动时间 1~2h。

(5) 电泳完毕，关闭电源，取出琼脂板，观察结果。

**【实验结果】**

在黑色背景上方，透过散射光线，首先观察 1 与 2 孔间（阳性对照组）、5 与 6 孔间（阴性对照组）的白色沉淀线是否出现；再看实验孔，如孔间未出现这样的沉淀线，则该待检血清为 HBsAg 阴性血清。阴性对照组不应出现沉淀线，否则实验无效。

**【注意事项】**

(1) 电泳时电流不宜过大，以免因发热使蛋白质变性或使凝胶断裂。

(2) 抗原与抗体的电极方向不能接反。

(3) 抗原与抗体的相对浓度要适当，抗原太浓或太稀时都不易出现沉淀线。

(4) 电泳所需时间与孔间距离有关，距离越大，电泳时间越长。

**【Materials and Equipment】**

(1) 1% ionic agar (Add the same amount of distilled water and 1% agar into pH8.6 barbitone buffer. Then the solution is filtered by absorbent cotton and sub-packaged, dissolved by heat before test).

(2) Anti-HBsAg antibody (diagnostic serum), HBsAg positive serum, testing serum, HBsAg negative serum, normal saline.

(3) Micropipettes and plastic tips, pipettes and rubber tips, slides, puncher and template.

(4) Electrophoresis tank, electrophoresis apparatus (Pour pH8.6 barbitone buffer in electrophoresis tank, cut filter paper at proper length and width which will be used to connect the slides to the buffer in the tank).

**【Procedures】**

(1) 4–5mL of melted 1% ionic agar is poured on the slide to make the agar slide.

(2) Punch wells according to the template after the agar slide has solidified. And use the micropipette to place anti-HBsAg antibody in the second, fourth and sixth wells, the testing serum in the third well, HBsAg positive serum in the first well as positive control and HBsAg negative serum in the fifth well as negative control. 10μL per well.

(3) Place the agar slide in the electrophoresis tank with the antigen in the cathode and antibody in the anode. Put one end of filter paper on the two sides of agar slide about 0.5cm away from the edge, and the other end of filter paper in the electrophoresis solution.

(4) Switch on the power supply to perform electrophoresis. The voltage, current and electrophoresis time depend on the performance of the equipment. In general, a voltage of 6V/cm, current of 20mA per slide, running time of 1–2h are used.

(5) After the run, switch off the power supply, take out the agar slide and observe the results.

**【Results】**

Against the black background, observe the white precipitation lines between the first and second wells (positive control group), the fifth and sixth wells (negative control group); then look at the test wells, if no precipitation line is observed, it means the testing serum would be HBsAg negative serum. Negative control group should not produce the precipitation line, otherwise, the test fails.

**【Attentions】**

(1) When running the electrophoresis, the current should be low so as to avoid the denaturation of protein and fracture of gel.

(2) The electrode direction of antigen and antibody can not be reversed.

(3) The relative concentration of antigen and antibody should be appropriate, or it is not easy to form precipitation lines.

(4) Distance between wells show a linear relationship to electrophoresis time, the farther the distance is, the longer the time of electrophoresis is.

## 四、免疫电泳实验

【实验目的】

掌握免疫电泳实验的原理、应用及结果分析，了解其基本操作方法。

【实验原理】

免疫电泳实验（immunoelectrophoresis test）是凝胶电泳与双向免疫扩散相结合的一种免疫学分析技术，将待检的可溶性物质在琼脂板上进行电泳分离，通过电泳能够把混合物中的各种不同成分分离开来，从而形成不同的区带。当电泳完毕后，加入相应抗血清，置湿盒内让其进行双向扩散，即可在相应位置上形成肉眼可见的乳白色的特异性沉淀线。每条沉淀线代表一组抗原抗体复合物，并可根据其迁移率与抗体所出现的特异反应进行鉴定。根据沉淀线的数量、位置及形状，可以分析标本中所含成分的性质（图 5）。

免疫电泳实验实际上分为两个步骤：

(1) 琼脂平板电泳将待检抗原物质在琼脂板上进行电泳分离。由于各种可溶性蛋白分子的大小、质量与所带电荷不同，在电场的作用下，其带电分子的运动速度也不相同，因此能够把混合物中的各种不同成分因电泳迁移率的不同而彼此分开。

(2) 琼脂扩散电泳后，在琼脂槽内加入相应的抗血清，进行免疫扩散，当已分离的各抗原成分与抗体在扩散中相遇且比例适合时，可形成肉眼可见的特异性沉淀线。根据沉淀线的数量及位置即可分析抗原的组成成分及其性质。

本实验以人血清 Ig 的分离鉴定为例来介绍免疫电泳实验。

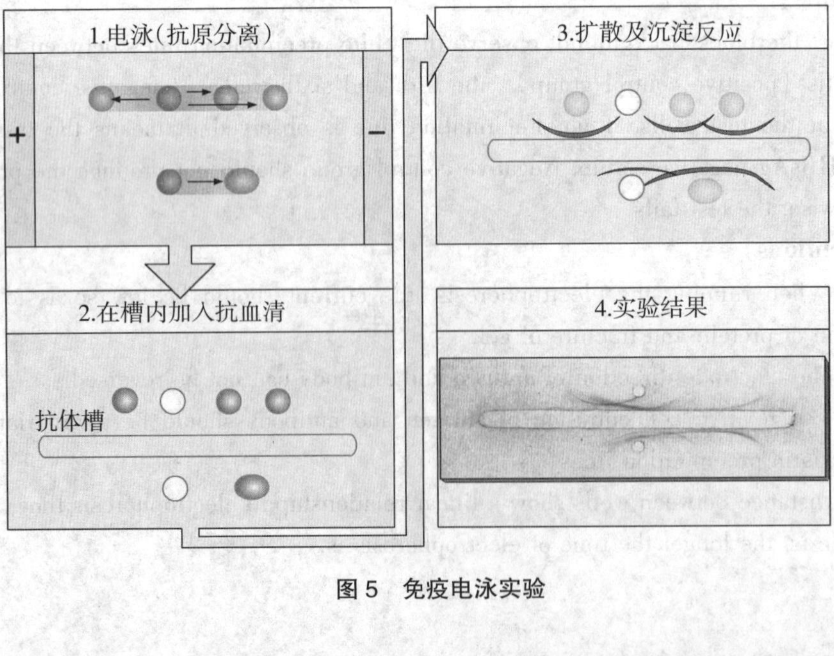


图 5 免疫电泳实验

## ⅳ. Immunoelectrophoresis Test

**【Aim】**

To master the principle of immunoelectrophoresis test, its application and the analysis of its results, be familiar with its basic methods of operation.

**【Principle】**

Immunoelectrophoresis test is an immunological analysis technique combining gel electrophoresis with double immunodiffusion. The testing soluble substances are separated by electrophoresis on the agar slide, and it is able to put the various components of the mixture separated and form some different zones. After electrophoresis stops, add the corresponding antibody serum, place the agar slide in moist chamber for double immunodiffusion. And you can observe visible milky specific precipitation lines, in the corresponding positions. Each line represents a group of antigen-antibody complexes and can be identified by its mobility and the specific reaction of the antibody. According to the amount of the precipitation lines, their locations and shapes, we can analyze the nature of the components in the samples (Figure 5).

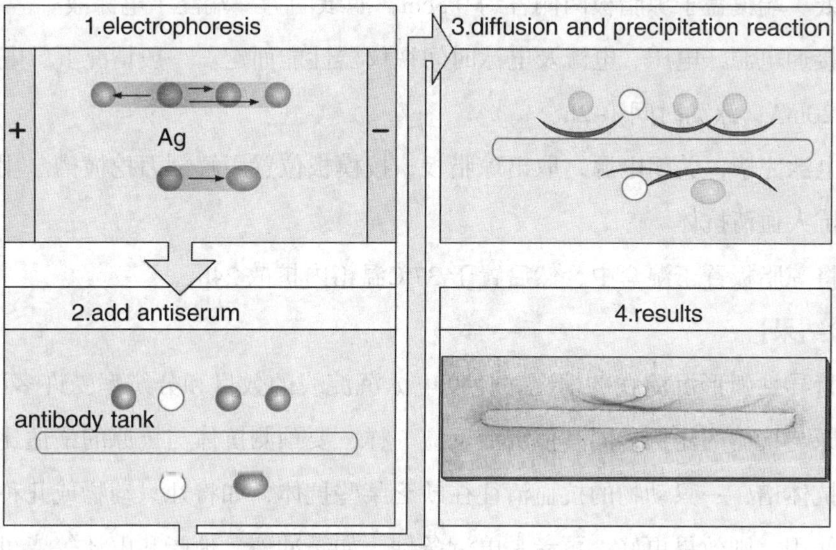


Figure 5 Immunoelectrophoresis Test

Immunoelectrophoresis test includes two steps:

(1) The antigen substances being tested on the agar slide are seperated by electrophoresis. Since the size, quality and the electric charge of a variety of soluble proteins are different, the speed of movement of charged molecules is also different in the electric field, it is possible to let the different components of the mixture separated due to different electrophoretic mobilities.

(2) After the agar diffusion electrophoresis, add the corresponding antiserum into the agar tank and make it diffuse. When the separated antigen meets with the corresponding

【实验器材】

(1) 巴比妥缓冲液（0.05mol/L，pH8.6）。

(2) 1.5%琼脂（用上述缓冲液配制）。

(3) 待检血清。

(4) 人 IgG（1mg/mL）。

(5) 兔抗人血清抗体。

(6) 载玻片、打孔器（3mm）、电泳仪、电泳槽、万用电表等。

【实验方法】

(1) 将融化的 1%离子琼脂倾注于玻片上制成琼脂板。

(2) 待琼脂板冷却凝固后，按照模板于挖槽线上下两侧各打一个孔，并分别用微量加样器加入待检血清及人 IgG15μL。

(3) 将琼脂板置于电泳槽内，注意电泳标本应放在负极“-”一侧，并将已浸透缓冲液的滤纸一端覆盖于琼脂板两侧各约 0.5cm，滤纸的另一端浸于电泳液中。

(4) 接通电源，电压、电流及电泳时间视仪器性能而定。一般情况下，电压 6V/cm，电流每板 20mA，泳动时间 1~2h。

(5) 电泳完毕，关闭电源，取出琼脂板，按模板位置用解剖刀挖横槽。用特制尖吸管加入兔抗人血清抗体。

(6) 将琼脂板置于湿盒中，然后置于 37℃温箱内扩散 24h。

【实验结果】

观察特异性弧形沉淀线的情况，免疫电泳沉淀线的数目和分辨率受许多因素影响。首先是抗原与抗体的比例，同其他沉淀反应一样，要预测抗体与抗原的最适比；其次是抗血清的抗体谱，一只动物的抗血清往往缺乏某些抗体，如将几只动物或几种动物的抗血清混合使用，则效果更好；再者是电泳条件，如缓冲液、琼脂和电泳等皆可直接影响沉淀线的分辨率。

【注意事项】

(1) 操作时动作要轻巧，挖槽时要注意平行整齐，加入抗体时不要外溢。

(2) 电泳后，可直接观察，也可染色观察。无色标本要在黑色背景下，用斜射光观察。

(3) 搭桥应完全紧密接触，以免因电流不均而发生沉淀线歪曲现象。

(4) 抗血清虽然含有所有抗原物质的相应抗体，但抗体效价有高有低，抗血清中必须含有足够的抗体，才能与被检样品中的所有抗原物质发生沉淀反应。因此要适当考虑抗原孔径的大小和抗体槽的距离。

antibody, they can produce visible specific precipitation lines in the appropriate proportion. We can analyze the nature and component of the antigen according to the precipitation lines' number and location.

This test takes human Ig serum's separation and identification as an example to introduce immunoelectrophoresis test.

**【Materials and Equipment】**

(1) Barbitone buffer (0.05mol/L, pH8.6).

(2) 1.5% agar (made by the above buffer).

(3) Testing serum.

(4) Human IgG (1mg/mL).

(5) Anti-human serum antibody produced in rabbit.

(6) Slides, puncher (diameter=3mm), electrophoresis apparatus, electrophoresis tank, avometer, etc.

**【Procedures】**

(1) Pour the 1% ionic agar which is melt on the slide to make the agar slide.

(2) After the agar is solidified, punch one well at both sides of the chamfer line according to the template. And add testing serum and human IgG respectively into wells by micropipettes, 15μL per well.

(3) Place the agar slide in the electrophoresis tank with the samples in the cathode side. And put one end of the filter paper on both sides of the agar slide about 0.5cm away from the edge, and the other end of the filter paper in the electrophoresis solution.

(4) Switch on the power supply to perform electrophoresis. The voltage, current and electrophoresis time depend on the performance of the equipment. In general, a voltage of 6V/cm, current of 20mA per slide and running time of 1–2h are used.

(5) After the run, switch off the power supply, take out the agar slide, and according to the template's location, use a scalpel to dig a horizontal slot. Add anti-human serum antibody produced in rabbit with special pipette in it.

(6) Place the agar slide in moist chamber, then put the moist chamber in 37℃ thermostat for 24h.

**【Results】**

Observe the specific curved precipitation lines, the number and resolution of the precipitation lines during immunoelectrophoresis are affected by many factors. The first is the ratio of antigen and antibody. As other precipitation reactions, it has to predict the optimal ratio of antibody and antigen. The second is antibody repertoire of antiserum. Antiserum of one animal is often lack of certain antibodies. If we mix antiserums from a few animals or several kinds of animals, the results would be better. The third is that the electrophoresis conditions can directly affect the resolution of the precipitation lines, such as buffers, agar and electrophoresis, etc.

**【Attentions】**

(1) Operation should be gentle, and slots should be in parallel. Do not overflow when

## 五、火箭电泳实验

【实验目的】

熟悉火箭电泳实验的原理和方法，了解该技术的临床应用。

【实验原理】

火箭电泳又称电泳实验免疫分析，是单向免疫扩散和电泳技术结合的实验。在电场作用下，抗原在含定量抗体的琼脂板中泳动，两者比例合适时，形成火箭似的锥形沉淀线，锥形沉淀线的高度与抗原量呈线性关系（成正比关系）（图 6），因此用本实验可以测定样品中抗原的含量。此法与单向免疫扩散法比较，优点是精密度较高、耗时较短，但不足之处是操作技术复杂，影响因素较多。

【实验器材】

（1）抗原：待测人血清标本及已知的纯化人 IgG 样品。

（2）抗体：兔抗人 IgG 血清。

（3）琼脂：用 pH8.6 的巴比妥缓冲液配制的 1.5%琼脂，溶化后于 60℃保温。

（4）2.2mol/L 甲醛液。

（5）器材：电泳仪、电泳槽、玻片、吸管、微量加样器、打孔器等。

【实验方法】

（1）先将 1.5%琼脂糖凝胶于沸水浴中加热溶化，保温于 52℃水浴中，加入适量兔抗人 IgG 血清，当抗体浓度为 0.75%~1%时，迅速混匀，倾注于水平放置的清洁干燥的玻板上，待其冷却。

（2）打孔：孔径 3mm，孔间距 5mm。

（3）抗原的醛化：

①先将血清标本和已知的纯化人 IgG 样品作不同浓度稀释。前者稀释为 1:40，后者稀释为 1:10、1:20、1:40、1:80。

②分别取 0.3mL 样品和 0.2mL 2.2mol/L 甲醛液置于一列小试管内，混匀，放入 37℃温箱 5min，进行醛化。

（4）每孔内加入不同稀释度的标准抗原及待检抗原，每孔 10μL。

（5）电泳抗原端接负极，电压 3V/cm，电泳 6~8h。

adding the antibody.

(2) After electrophoresis, we can observe the result directly, or after staining. Observe the colorless samples against a black background under slanting light.

(3) Salt bridge should be completely attached, so as to avoid the occurrence of distorted precipitation line due to uneven current.

(4) Although antiserum contains the corresponding antibodies of all antigens, antibodies' titers are different, antiserum must contain sufficient antibodies, so as to react with all antigens and produce precipitation. Therefore, the diameters of the antigen wells and the distance of the antibody slots should be considered.

## V. Rocket Electrophoresis Test

**【Aim】**

To master the principle and methods of rocket electrophoresis test. To know its clinical application.

**【Principle】**

Rocket electrophoresis, also called electrophoresis immunology analysis, is an experiment combining single immunodiffusion with electrophoresis. In the electric field, the antigen runs in agar slide which contains certain amount of antibodies. When their proportion is proper, a cone precipitation line which looks like a rocket will be formed. The height of the cone precipitation line shows a linear relationship to the amount of antigen (Figure 6). Therefore, the antigen content in the sample can be determined in this test. Compared to single immunodiffusion, it has the advantages of high precision, shorter time-consuming, and the disadvantages are that the operation technique is complex and it is influenced by many factors.

**【Materials and Equipment】**

(1) Antigen: the testing human serum samples, the known purified human IgG samples.

(2) Antibody: anti-human IgG serum produced in rabbit.

(3) Agar: 1.5% agar which is made by pH8.6 barbitone buffer, preserved at 60℃ after being dissolved.

(4) 2. 2mol/L formaldehyde solution.

(5) Equipment: electrophoresis apparatus, electrophoresis tank, slides, suckers, micropipettes, puncher, etc.

**【Procedures】**

(1) Firstly, melt the 1.5% agarose gel in a boiling water bath and preserve it in 52℃ water bath, add appropriate amount of anti-human IgG serum produced in rabbit, when the concentration of antibody is between 0.75% and 1%, rapidly mix and pour it on a clean and dry slide, let it cool down.

(2) Punch wells, with the diameter of 3mm and the distance between two wells being 5mm.

(3) Hydroformylation of antigen:

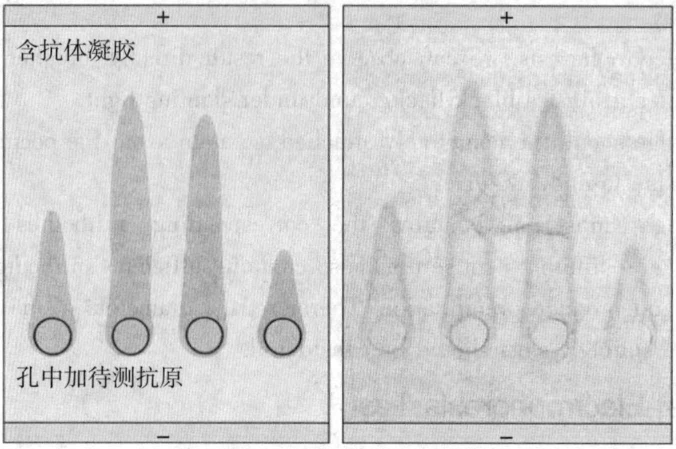


图 6　火箭电泳实验

【实验结果】

(1) 琼脂板上出现不同高度的沉淀峰，形似火箭。

(2) 制作标准曲线：以沉淀峰的高度为纵坐标，抗原浓度为横坐标。根据测得的待检抗原峰的高度查标准曲线，即知待检抗原浓度。

【注意事项】

(1) 电泳后可直接观察，也可干燥后染色观察。

(2) 低电压、低离子强度、较长电泳时间会使效果更好。

(3) 加样后应及时电泳。

① Firstly dilute serum samples at 1: 40, and known human IgG samples at 1: 10, 1: 20, 1: 40, 1: 80 respectively.

② Place 0.3mL of each sample and 0.2mL 2.2mol/L formaldehyde solution in a row of small tubes, mix well and incubate in 37℃ thermostat for 5min for hydroformylation.

(4) Add standard antigens of different dilutions and testing antigens into wells, 10μL per well.

(5) Connect antigen end with the cathode, the voltage is 3V/cm, run electrophoresis for 6–8h.

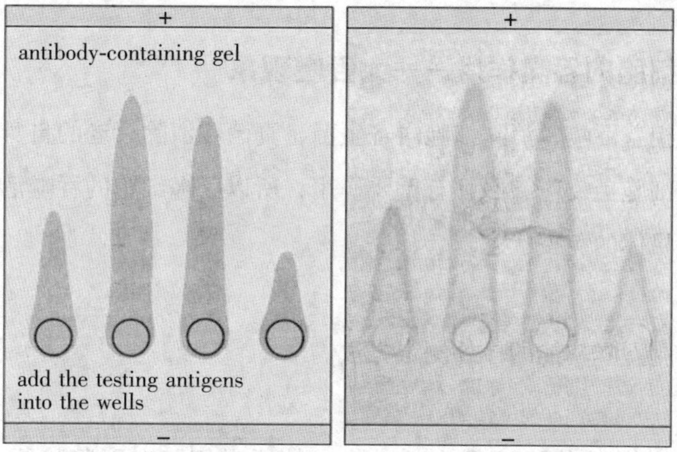


Figure 6 Rocket Electrophoresis Test

【Results】

(1) Precipitation peaks of different heights appear on the agar slide, their shapes are like rockets.

(2) Draw standard curve: use the heights of precipitation peaks as ordinate, the concentration of antigens as abscissa. The concentration of the testing antigen can be calculated based on the height of precipitation peak of the testing antigen according to the standard curve.

【Attentions】

(1) After electrophoresis, we can observe directly or after being stained.

(2) With lower voltage, lower ionic strength and longer electrophoresis time, the results will be better.

(3) After adding the samples, electrophoresis should start in time.

# 实验三 吞噬功能检测

## 一、巨噬细胞的吞噬作用——大吞噬现象

巨噬细胞承担着吞噬、消除细胞内寄生菌、真菌和清除衰老的自身细胞的职能，它在特异性体液或细胞免疫应答中都有重要作用，所以巨噬细胞的吞噬消化功能，在一定程度上可以反映机体的免疫状态。

**【实验目的】**

熟悉巨噬细胞吞噬功能的体外测定方法。

**【实验原理】**

利用注入腹腔的淀粉溶液作为刺激物，使巨噬细胞向腹腔移行，再将鸡红细胞（CRBC）注入小鼠腹腔。巨噬细胞可借助细胞表面的免疫识别受体或直接吞噬鸡红细胞而将其消化。通过显微镜观察该吞噬现象，计算吞噬百分率和吞噬指数，可判断巨噬细胞的吞噬功能。

**【实验器材】**

（1）小鼠、PBS 缓冲液、5%淀粉溶液、2%鸡红细胞悬液、瑞氏染液。

（2）剪刀、镊子、注射器、尖吸管及橡皮吸头、小试管、载玻片、普通光学显微镜、镜油、擦镜纸等。

**【实验方法】**

（1）实验准备：用无菌注射器吸取 5%淀粉溶液 2mL，注射于小鼠腹腔内。

（2）3 天后，往小鼠腹腔内注射 2%鸡红细胞悬液 2mL，让其活动 1h。

（3）将小鼠用颈椎脱臼法处死，解剖暴露腹腔，于腹腔靠上部位，用镊子轻轻夹起腹膜，将腹膜剪一个小口，用尖吸管注入 2~3mL 预温的 PBS 缓冲液，同时用手反复揉搓腹腔 1~2min，以便尽可能多地冲洗出小鼠腹腔内的巨噬细胞。

（4）用尖吸管吸取腹腔液，置于洁净试管内。用滴管吸出腹腔液滴加在玻片上，每片约 0.2mL。把这些玻片放入 37℃温箱中孵育 30min。

# III. Phagocytosis Test

## i. The Phagocytosis of Macrophage—Big Phagocytosis Phenomenon

The macrophages have the ability of phagocytizing, eliminating parasitic bacteria, fungi and aged cells, which makes them important in specific humoral and cellular immune responses. So the digestive function of macrophages, to a certain extent, can reflect the body's immune status.

**【Aim】**

Get familiar with the determination method of the phagocytosis of macrophages in vitro.

**【Principle】**

Using starch solution injected in mouse abdominal cavity as a stimulant, make macrophages move to abdominal cavity, then inject chicken red blood cells (CRBC) into abdominal cavity. Macrophages can phagocytize chicken red blood cells and digest them directly or use the immune on the surface of the cells to recognize receptors. Use microscope to observe this phenomenon, calculating the percentage and index of phagocytosis can determine the phagocytosis of macrophage.

**【Materials and Equipment】**

(1) Mouse, PBS buffer, 5% starch solution, 2% chicken red blood cells suspension, Wright's stain.

(2) Scissors, tweezers, syringes, pipettes and rubber tips, small tube, slides, ordinary optical microscope, immersion oil, lens paper, etc.

**【Procedures】**

(1) Preparation: use sterile syringes to inject 2mL 5% starch solution into mouse abdominal cavity.

(2) Three days later, inject 2mL 2% chicken red blood cells suspension into mouse abdominal cavity, let it be active for 1h.

(3) Kill the mouse by cervical dislocation, then expose its abdominal cavity. Clip up peritoneum of the upper part of abdominal cavity gently by tweezers, and cut them into a bite size, inject 2–3mL pre-warmed PBS buffer by pipette, at the same time rubbing abdominal cavity repeatedly for 1–2min by hand, so as to flush out the mouse's peritoneal macrophage as much as possible.

(5) 取出玻片，用 pH6.4 的 PBS 缓冲液轻轻冲洗玻片。巨噬细胞、中性粒细胞等吞噬细胞在孵育过程中已吸附在玻片上，轻轻冲洗不掉，其他非吞噬细胞则大部分被冲洗掉。自然干燥。

(6) 瑞氏染色：瑞氏染液 2~3 滴，染 1min，直接滴加蒸馏水 6~8 滴，染 6min，以蒸馏水冲洗。吸水纸吸干，油镜下观察巨噬细胞吞噬鸡红细胞现象。

**【实验结果】**

观察巨噬细胞对鸡红细胞的吞噬现象，计算吞噬百分比，即每 100 个吞噬细胞所吞噬的鸡红细胞数量。也可用吞噬指数表示，即将 100 个吞噬细胞所吞噬的鸡红细胞的总数除以 100。吞噬百分比和吞噬指数一般是平行的。吞噬百分比和吞噬指数都用于表示吞噬细胞的功能。

用油镜查找观察巨噬细胞 200 个。鸡红细胞为有核红细胞，经瑞氏染液染色后，胞浆呈粉红色，核呈紫蓝色。查找观察到的巨噬细胞，有的吞噬了鸡红细胞，有的未吞噬鸡红细胞，都应列入查找对象及计算范围。应注意区分鸡红细胞是真正被吞噬还是仅黏附于巨噬细胞表面。查找观察有吞噬作用的巨噬细胞数。被吞噬的鸡红细胞尚未被消化者，胞浆和核都很清晰；刚开始消化的，胞浆色变浅，界线不清；胞浆被消化者可仅留下紫色的核；再进一步消化时，可能只看到浅紫色的核轮廓。这些都应列入被吞噬的鸡红细胞数。

**【注意事项】**

(1) 向小鼠腹腔注射时不要刺伤内脏。

(2) 如小鼠腹腔液过少，可向腹腔注入适量生理盐水揉动后再取。

(3) 剪开小鼠腹腔时应避免出血，否则将影响实验结果。

(4) 必须掌握好吞噬作用的时间，时间过长，被吞噬的鸡红细胞可能被消化，时间过短，则未被吞噬。

(5) 涂片的薄厚要适当，否则影响计数。

(4) Transfer the peritoneal fluid by pipette into a clean tube. Drop the peritoneal fluid on the slides by dropper, about 0.2mL per slide. Put the slides in 37℃ thermostat for 30 minutes.

(5) Take out the slides and wash them with pH6.4 PBS buffer gently. Macrophages, neutrophils and other phagocytes in the incubation process have attached on the slides, which can't be rinsed off, other non-phagocytic cells are mostly rinsed off. Then let the slides be naturally dried.

(6) Wright's staining: Wright's stain 2–3 drops, dye 1min, directly add 6 to 8 drops of distilled water, dye 6min, rinse by distilled water. Dry out with blotting paper, under oil immersion lens observe the phenomenon of phagocytosis that macrophages phagocytize chicken red blood cells.

**【Results】**

When observe the phenomenon of phagocytosis that macrophages phagocytize chicken red blood cells, calculate phagocytic percentage, that is the number of chicken red blood cells being phagocytized in every 100 phagocytes. Phagocytic index can also be used, meaning the total number of chicken red blood cells being phagocytized in 100 phagocytes divided by 100. Phagocytic percentage and phagocytic index are generally parallel. Phagocytic percentage and phagocytic index are used to express the function of macrophages.

Use oil immersion lens to find 200 macrophages. Chicken red blood cell is a kind of nucleated red blood cell. After Wright's staining, cytoplasm is pink, with purple and blue nucleus. For the observation of macrophages, some swallowed chicken red blood cells, some not, all should be included as search object and calculation range. Pay attention to distinguish chicken red blood cells swallowed from those only adhere to the surface of the macrophage. Observe the phagocytic macrophages. Chicken red blood cells being phagocytized that have not yet been digested, the cytoplasm and nucleus are clear; at the beginning of digestion, cytoplasmic color turns lighter, without clear limit; cytoplasm can be digested and only leave the purple nucleus; with further digestion, it may only see light purple outline of nucleus. These should be listed in the number of chicken red blood cells being phagocytized to calculate the phagocytic percentage and phagocytic index.

**【Attentions】**

(1) Don't hurt the internal organs when injecting into mouse abdominal cavity.

(2) If the peritoneal fluid is not enough, you can inject appropriate amount of normal saline and rub before absorbing.

(3) Avoid bleeding when cutting the mouse abdominal cavity, otherwise it will affect the result.

(4) If it takes too long, the chicken red blood cells can be digested, while if the time is too short, chicken red blood cells will not be phagocytized, so the time of phagocytosis must be controlled.

(5) The thickness of smear should be appropriate, otherwise it will affect the count.

## 二、中性粒细胞的吞噬作用——小吞噬现象（体外法）

血液中的中性粒细胞通常被称为小吞噬细胞，有强大的吞噬和消化异物的功能，构成机体的天然抵抗力。在机体固有免疫和适应性免疫中发挥着重要的作用。对中性粒细胞的检测包括对其运动功能、吞噬功能和杀伤功能的测定。

**【实验目的】**

通过本实验的操作对中性粒细胞的非特异性吞噬功能加以验证，进一步理解中性粒细胞在免疫应答中的重要作用。

**【实验原理】**

血液中的中性粒细胞通过趋化、调理、吞入、杀伤和消化等步骤，清除病原体及衰老、死亡的细胞。中性粒细胞吞噬功能的测定可辅助诊断吞噬功能缺陷病。中性粒细胞具有吞噬细菌等异物颗粒的能力，在体外将中性粒细胞与细菌或其他异物颗粒共同孵育后，显微镜观察可见中性粒细胞内有细菌或异物颗粒。计算吞噬有细菌或异物颗粒的中性粒细胞数占中性粒细胞总数的百分比和每个中性粒细胞平均吞噬的细菌或异物颗粒数，可反映中性粒细胞的吞噬功能。该实验常用白色葡萄球菌作为中性粒细胞的吞噬物。

**【实验器材】**

（1）抗凝剂：3.8%柠檬酸钠。

（2）白色葡萄球菌孵育 18h 肉汤培养物（10 亿/毫升）

（3）清洁载玻片、无菌注射器，6 号、9 号针头及无菌肉汤。

（4）瑞氏染液、pH6.8 磷酸盐缓冲液（或蒸馏水）。

**【实验方法】**

（1）白色葡萄球菌孵育 18h 肉汤培养物（10 亿/毫升），加热至 100℃，15min，凉至 4℃备用。

（2）自静脉采血 0.2mL，置于含 0.2mL3.8%柠檬酸钠的小试管中，混匀，防止凝血。

（3）取白色葡萄球菌菌液 0.1mL，加入上述血液中混匀。

（4）37℃水浴静置孵育 30~40min。

（5）取出试管，用毛细管吸取白细胞层（即沉淀红细胞的表层），制成血膜，自然干燥。

（6）瑞氏染色。

①于玻片上滴加瑞氏染液数滴，覆盖血膜涂层，染色 1min。

②滴加与染液等量的蒸馏水（或 pH6.8 磷酸盐缓冲液）于玻片上，轻摇玻片，混匀

## ⅱ. Neutrophil Phagocytosis—Small Phagocytosis Phenomenon (In Vitro)

The neutrophil in the blood known as microphage has a strong phagocytosis and digestion of foreign materials that form the body's natural resistance. It plays an important role in the innate immunity and adaptive immunity. The detection of neutrophil includes the determination of its movement, phagocytosis and killing functions.

**【Aim】**

Through the experiment of nonspecific phagocytosis of neutrophils, understand the significant role of neutrophils in the immune response.

**【Principle】**

Through chemotaxis, opsonize, phagocytizing, killing and digesting, neutrophils in blood remove pathogens, aging and dead cells. The determination of neutrophil phagocytosis can assist in the diagnosis of dysphagocytosis. Neutrophils have the ability of phagocytizing bacteria and other foreign particles. After incubation with bacteria or other foreign particles together in vitro, neutrophils containing bacteria or foreign particles are observed with microscope. Calculate the percentage of neutrophils which phagocytize bacteria or foreign particles of the total number of neutrophils, and average number of bacteria or foreign particles phagocytized per neutrophil, which can reflect the phagocytosis of the neutrophils. The experiment often uses *S. albus* as bacteria being phagocytized by neutrophils.

**【Materials and Equipment】**

(1) Anticoagulant: 3.8% sodium citrate.

(2) 18h broth culture of *S. albus*(1 billion/mL)

(3) Clean slides, sterile syringe, 6, 9 needles and sterile broth.

(4) Wright's stain, pH6.8 phosphate buffer (or distilled water).

**【Procedures】**

(1) Heat 18h broth culture of *S. albus* (1 billion/mL) to 100℃ for 15min, then cool it down to 4℃ for later use.

(2) Collect 0.2mL venous blood, place it in a small tube containing 0.2mL 3.8% sodium citrate, blending to prevent blood clotting.

(3) Take 0.1mL *S. albus* liquid, add it in the above blood, blending.

(4) Incubate in 37℃ water bath for 30–40min.

(5) Take out the tube, using capillary to drain white blood cells layer (the surface layer of the precipitation of red blood cells), and make it into blood film, natural drying.

(6) Wright's staining.

①Add several drops of Wright's stain on the slide to cover blood film, dye for 1min.

②Drop the same amount of distilled water (or pH6.8 phosphate buffer) on the slide, shake the slide gently, blend and dye for 3–5min.

③Rinse with slow water, dry out with blotting paper, and observe under oil immersion lens.

染液，染 3~5min。

③流水缓慢冲洗，吸水纸吸干后用油镜观察。

**【实验结果】**

中性粒细胞的细胞核被染成深紫红色，核分 2~5 叶，细胞质被染成淡粉红色；白色葡萄球菌被染成深紫色。随机选取 100 个中性粒细胞，分别计算吞噬有细菌的吞噬细胞数和所吞噬的细菌总数，分别计算出吞噬百分比和吞噬指数。

**【Results】**

Nucleus of neutrophils is dyed into deep purple red, and divided into 2 –5 leaves, cytoplasm is dyed into light pink; *S. albus* is dyed into deep purple. Randomly choose 100 neutrophils, and count the number of neutrophils phagocytizing at least one bacterium and the total number of bacteria being phagocytized, respectively. Calculate the phagocytic percentage and phagocytic index.

# 实验四　小鼠脾细胞的制备

脾脏是体内最大的免疫器官，是各种成熟淋巴细胞定居的场所，其中B细胞约占脾淋巴细胞总数的60%,T细胞约占脾淋巴细胞总数的40%，还有少量NK细胞。由于小鼠脾细胞中含有T细胞、B细胞和NK细胞，因此，在科研工作中常用小鼠脾细胞来进行淋巴细胞功能的检测，比如T细胞增殖功能的检测、B细胞增殖功能的检测，NK细胞杀伤功能的检测等。本实验运用机械方法使脾细胞从脏器中分离出来。

**【实验目的】**

熟悉小鼠脾细胞的制备方法及其在科研工作中的实际应用。

**【实验原理】**

小鼠脾细胞中含有T细胞、B细胞和少量NK细胞，从小鼠脾细胞中获得上述细胞，可分别用于在体外检测小鼠的细胞免疫功能、体液免疫功能及NK细胞的杀伤功能。

**【实验器材】**

（1）6~8周龄昆明种小鼠，雌雄不限。

（2）75%酒精、碘酒、生理盐水、蒸馏水、红细胞裂解液（Tris-$NH_4Cl$）、0.05%锥兰染液，RPMI-1640培养液。

（3）解剖器械（眼科剪、眼科镊）、托盘、150mm直径玻璃平皿、100目不锈钢网、吸管、试管、水平离心机、试管架等。

**【实验方法】**

（1）用颈椎脱臼法处死小鼠，浸入75%的酒精中浸泡1~2分钟。

（2）小心剪开小鼠的腹部外皮，用大头针固定，撕开皮肤，暴露腹壁，可见长条状、紫红色的脏器，此即为脾脏。用镊子取出小鼠脾脏放在不锈钢网（100目）上，注意无菌操作。

（3）加入2mL RPMI-1640培养液，然后用注射器活塞轻轻研磨小鼠脾脏。

（4）加入2mL RPMI-1640培养液，冲洗网上残余细胞。

# IV. The Preparation of Mouse Splenocyte

Spleen is the body's largest immune organ and is the place that all sorts of mature lymphocytes settled, while the B cells account for about 60% of the total number of splenic lymphocytes, T cells account for about 40% of the total number of splenic lymphocytes, and NK cells are in a small amount. Because mouse splenocytes contain T cells, B cells and NK cells, we often use mouse splenocytes in the scientific research work to test the function of lymphocytes, such as proliferation test of T/B cells and the test of the killing ability of NK cells, etc. This experiment using mechanical method makes the splenocyte isolated from the viscera.

**【Aim】**

Get familiar with the preparation of mouse splenocyte and the actual application in scientific research work.

**【Principle】**

Mouse splenocytes contain T cells, B cells and a small amount of NK cells, the cells from mouse splenocytes can be respectively used for in vitro detection of cellular immune function, humoral immune function in mouse and NK cells' killing ability.

**【Materials and Equipment】**

(1) 6–8 weeks of Kunming mouse of either gender.

(2) 75% alcohol, iodine, normal saline, distilled water, red blood cell lysis buffer (Tris-$NH_4Cl$), 0.05% trypan-blue, RPMI-1640 culture medium.

(3) Dissecting instruments (eye scissors, eye tweezers), tray, 150mm diameter glass plate, 100-mesh stainless steel wire mesh, straw, test tube, horizontal centrifuge, test tube rack, etc.

**【Procedures】**

(1) Kill the mouse by cervical dislocation, immerse it in 75% alcohol for 1–2 minutes.

(2) Carefully cut the abdominal skin of mouse, fixe it with a pin, tear the skin, expose the abdominal wall, you can see long, purple viscera, which is the spleen. Use the tweezer to take out the mouse spleen in a stainless steel wire mesh (100-mesh), pay attention to the aseptic operation.

(3) Add 2mL RPMI-1640 culture medium, and then gently grind mouse spleen with syringe piston.

（5）将全部液体收集到离心管中，1 500rpm 离心 10 分钟，去上清液。

（6）加入 2mL RPMI-1640 培养液，1 500rpm 离心 10 分钟，去上清液。

（7）加入 2mL Tris-$NH_4Cl$，1 分钟消化红细胞，再加入 6mL RPMI-1640 培养液，1 500rpm 离心 10 分钟，去上清液。

（8）加入 1mL RPMI-1640 培养液，计算脾细胞数量。

（9）取 0.1mL 细胞悬液与等量 0.05%锥兰染液混匀，5~10min 后取一滴滴于血球计数板上，高倍镜下计算四个大方格内的细胞总数。死细胞被染成蓝色，体积较大且无光泽；活细胞体积较小而透明，不着色。按下列公式求出脾细胞总数：

脾细胞浓度（细胞数／毫升悬液）=（四个大方格内细胞总数／4）$\times 10^4 \times$ 稀释倍数

**【实验结果】**

（1）观察脾脏结构是否完整，称重。

（2）细胞计数时用 0.05%锥兰染液染色后观察，活细胞比例应在 90%以上。根据计数结果，将脾细胞悬液配成实验所需浓度。

**【注意事项】**

（1）使用低渗法溶解脾细胞中的红细胞时，低渗状态不能超过 1min，否则会影响所分离脾细胞的活性。

（2）因为分离出的脾细胞在后续实验中还要继续培养，故操作过程要严格无菌；要在冰浴中制备脾细胞，以尽量避免细胞死亡带来的误差。

（3）手术器械除术前高压灭菌外，也可将手术器械浸泡在 95%酒精中，使用前取出器械，在酒精灯上烧灼去除酒精，即可保证无菌，此法较为简便。

(4) Add 2mL RPMI-1640 culture medium, flushing residual cells on the mesh.

(5) Collect all the liquid to a centrifuge tube, centrifuge at the speed of 1,500 RPM for 10 minutes and discard the supernatant.

(6) Add 2mL RPMI-1640 culture medium, centrifuge at the speed of 1,500 RPM for 10 minutes and discard the supernatant.

(7) Add 2mL Tris-$NH_4Cl$, sit for 1min to lyze the red blood cells, add 6mL RPMI-1640 culture medium, centrifuge at the speed of 1,500 RPM for 10min and discard the supernatant.

(8) Add 1mL RPMI-1640 culture medium, and count the cells.

(9) Take 0.1mL cell suspension and mix with 0.1mL 0.05% trypan-blue, take a drop on the blood counting chamber after 5-10min, count the total number of cells within the four big squares under high power lens. Dead cells are dyed blue, large and without luster; living cells are smaller and transparent, with no color. According to the following formula to calculate the total number of splenocytes:

Concentration of splenocytes (number of cells/mL of suspension) = (total cells within the four big squares / 4)$\times 10^4\times$dilution ratio。

**【Results】**

(1) Observe the spleen to see whether it is complete or not. Then weigh it.

(2) Count the cells which are dyed by 0.05% trypan-blue. Living cells should count for above 90%. According to the results of the count, prepare the suspension of splenocytes into the solution with the concentration needed for the experiment.

**【Attentions】**

(1) When use low osmotic pressure method to dissolve the red blood cells in splenocytes, the state of low osmotic pressure cannot exceed 1min, otherwise it will affect the viability of splenocytes.

(2) Because in the subsequent experiments, it will continue to culture isolated splenocytes, strict aseptic operation is required; splenocyte preparation should be placed in an ice bath to avoid cell death.

(3) In addition to autoclave, operation instruments can also be soaked in 95% alcohol. Take out before using, burn to remove alcohol in alcohol lamp, which can ensure sterilization. This method is relatively simple.

# 实验五　溶血空斑实验

【实验目的】

掌握溶血空斑实验的原理、操作方法及其检测的临床意义。

【实验原理】

溶血空斑实验，又称空斑形成细胞（plaque forming cell，PFC）实验，是一种体外检测抗体形成细胞的方法。将经绵羊红细胞（sheep red blood cells, SRBC）免疫的小鼠脾细胞（含有抗体形成细胞）与一定量的绵羊红细胞和补体混合孵育。PFC 所分泌的抗体和绵羊红细胞结合形成抗原抗体复合物，在补体作用下可使绵羊红细胞溶解，在特制的小室内形成肉眼可见的溶血空斑。一个空斑即代表一个抗体形成细胞（图 7）。本实验可作为机体体液免疫状态的指标，研究免疫增强和抑制药物对机体免疫功能的影响等特异性指标。目前所用的 PFC 检查法有：琼脂固相法、单层细胞法、小室液相法。本书介绍小室液相法。

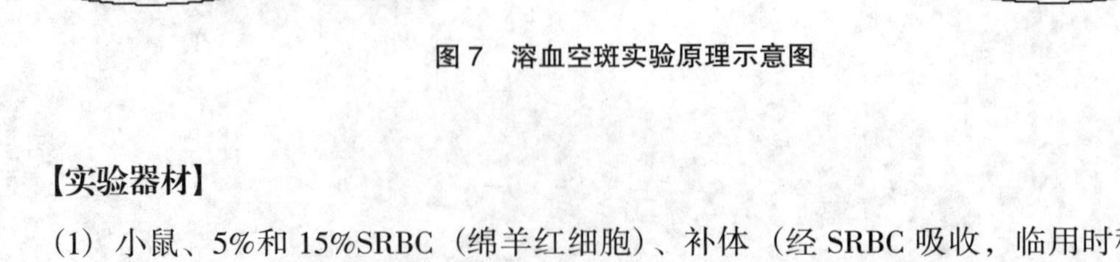


图 7　溶血空斑实验原理示意图

【实验器材】

（1）小鼠、5%和 15%SRBC（绵羊红细胞）、补体（经 SRBC 吸收，临用时稀释成 1:6 浓度）、Hank's 液。

# V. Hemolytic Plaque Formation Test

【Aim】

To master the principle, procedure and clinical significance of the hemolytic plaque formation test.

【Principle】

Hemolytic plaque formation test, which is also called plaque forming cell (PFC) test, is a method used to detect antibody-forming cells in vitro. Splenocytes obtained from the mouse immunized with sheep red blood cells (SRBC) are incubated with SRBC and complement together. Antibody produced by PFC combines with sheep red blood cells, forming an antigen-antibody complex. The complement makes sheep red blood cells dissolve, forming hemolytic plaques in special chambers, which is visible by naked eyes. One hemolytic plaque corresponds to one antibody-forming cell (Figure 7). The test can be used to study the state of humoral immunity, the efficiency of drugs for immune suppression or enhancement. The test can be performed with agar solid-phase method, monolayer cell method and chamber liquid-phase method. We use chamber liquid-phase method here.

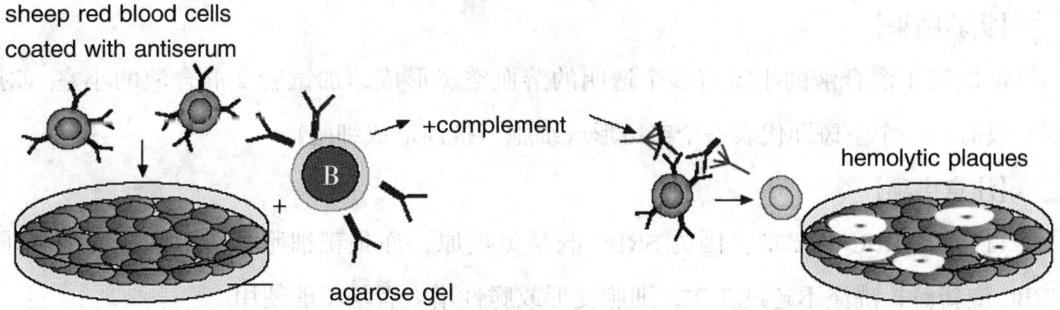


Figure 7 Principle of Hemolytic Plaque Formation Test

【Materials and Equipment】

(1) Mouse, 5% and 15% sheep red blood cells, complement (absorbed by sheep red blood cells, dilute into 1:6 when be used), Hank's solution.

(2) Test tubes, 1mL pipettes, clean and grease-free slides, paraffin, micropipettes and tips, 100-mesh stainless steel wire mesh, nylon mesh, plates, double-faced masking tape,

(2) 试管、1mL 吸量管、洁净无脂载玻片、石蜡、微量加样器及吸头、100 目不锈钢网、尼龙网、平皿、双面胶带、注射器。

(3) 37℃孵箱、离心机、普通光学显微镜。

**【实验方法】**

(1) 免疫小鼠脾细胞悬液的制备：取 0.4mL 5%SRBC 注射小鼠腹腔，4 天后用颈椎脱臼法将其处死，取出脾脏置于 100 目不锈钢网上，在已加入 7mL Hank's 液的平皿中研磨，用尼龙网过滤至试管，混匀，1 000r/min 离心 10min。用 Hank's 液洗两次，最后将沉淀的脾细胞重悬于 1mL Hank's 液中，即为浓度约 $1\times10^7$/mL 的脾细胞悬液。

(2) 制作小室：取洁净无脂载玻片（75mm×25mm）两张，在载玻片两端和中间各粘一条双面胶带，将两张同样的载玻片紧密地粘在一起，即形成两个小室。将此双层玻片的一侧长边浸入融化的石蜡池中以封闭小室的一边（无须浸入过深，以能封闭小室边缘为准）。

(3) 制备小室灌注混合液：

试管 1：取 $1\times10^7$/mL 脾细胞悬液 50μL、15%SRBC 50μL、1:6 补体 50μL、Hank's 液 250μL。

试管 2：取 $1\times10^7$/mL 脾细胞悬液 50μL、15%SRBC 50μL、Hank's 液 300μL。

混匀后，用微量加样器分别取上述两支试管中的混合液灌注两个小室（尽量避免产生气泡），蜡封，做好标记，平放于玻片盘内，置于 37℃孵箱内孵育 45min~1h 后观察结果。

**【实验结果】**

加试管 1 混合液的小室有多个透明的溶血空斑形成，加试管 2 混合液的小室（对照）没有。一个空斑即代表一个空斑形成细胞（抗体形成细胞）。

**【注意事项】**

(1) 对 SRBC 的要求：因为 SRBC 既是免疫原，亦是靶细胞和指示细胞，故要求 SRBC 应新鲜，洗涤不超过 3 次，细胞变形或脆性增大者均不能使用。

(2) 采取免疫脾的时间：以免疫后第四天取脾为宜，过早或过晚空斑都形成极少。

(3) 为了保持脾细胞的活力，制备脾细胞过程中所用的 Hank's 液，最好临用时方从 4℃冰箱中取出，或整个操作过程应在冰浴中进行。

(4) 孵育时，要把握好温度。小室注入混合液时不要留有气泡，小室边缘须封严。

syringe.

(3) 37℃ incubator, centrifuge, the ordinary optical microscope.

**【Procedures】**

(1) Prepare immunized mouse splenocyte suspension: Inject the mouse with 0. 4mL 5% sheep red blood cells via abdomen, kill the mouse by cervical dislocation 4 days later, take out its spleen on 100-mesh stainless steel wire mesh and grind it in a plate with 7mL Hank's solution. Filter the mixture with nylon mesh, collect the suspension into a tube, mix and centrifuge it at the speed of 1, 000r/min for 10min. Then wash the cells with Hank's solution for 2 times. At last, add 1mL Hank's solution into the cells, the concentration of the splenocyte suspension should be approximately $1\times10^7$ /mL.

(2) Prepare the chambers: Prepare two slides (75mm×25mm) which are clean and free of grease. Carefully lay a strip of double-faced masking tape at both ends and the center of the slides. Stick two slides together to form two chambers. Immerse the long side of the double slides into melted paraffin to close one side of the chambers (suitable depth is needed).

(3) Prepare the mixture for perfusing the chambers:

Tube 1: Add 50μL $1\times10^7$/mL splenocyte suspensation, 50μL 15% sheep red blood cells, 50μl complement diluted to 1:6 and 250μL Hank's solution to the tube.

Tube 2: Add 50μL $1\times10^7$/mL splenocyte suspensation, 50μL 15% sheep red blood cells and 300μL Hank's solution to the tube.

Mix them well, take the above mixture of each tube to perfuse each chamber(try to avoid forming bubble) by using micropipettes , close each side with paraffin, mark and lay them in the slide plate, incubate in 37℃ incubator for 45min to 1h, and then observe the result.

**【Results】**

Numbers of transparent hemolytic plaques should be seen in the chamber perfused by mixture of tube 1, non in the other. One hemolytic plaque corresponds to one antibody-forming cell.

**【Attentions】**

(1) Requirements of sheep red blood cells: Because they are immunogen, as well as target cells and indicator cells, the sheep red blood cells should be fresh and can not be washed for more than three times. Those deformed and brittle cells can not be used.

(2) The time of taking the immunized spleen: It is appropriate to take the immunized spleen 4 days later, either too late or too early will lead to less plaques forming.

(3) To keep the vitality of the splenocytes, Hank's solution should be taken out of 4℃ refrigerator, or all the procedures are taken in ice bath.

(4) Keep at appropriate temperature when incubate. Make sure there is no bubble in the chambers. Each side of the chamber should be closed completely.

# 实验六 E 玫瑰花环形成实验

**【实验目的】**

熟悉 E 玫瑰花环形成实验的原理、方法及应用。

**【实验原理】**

正常人外周血 T 淋巴细胞表面具有能和绵羊红细胞（SRBC）膜上的糖蛋白相结合的受体，称为 E 受体（即 CD2），是人 T 淋巴细胞所特有的表面标志。E 受体在体外一定条件下，能与绵羊等动物的红细胞结合，形成以 T 淋巴细胞为中心，红细胞环绕在其周围的 E 玫瑰花环。已证实 90%以上的 T 淋巴细胞及部分单核巨噬细胞具有 E 受体。当 T 淋巴细胞与 SRBC 混合后，SRBC 便附于 T 淋巴细胞表面，呈花环状。通过玫瑰花环形成检查 T 淋巴细胞的方法，称为 E 玫瑰花环形成实验。根据形成花环的多少，可测得 T 淋巴细胞的数目，从而间接了解机体细胞免疫功能状态，判断疾病的预后，考核药物疗效等。

本实验可作为人外周血 T 淋巴细胞的鉴定和计数，形成 E 花环后的 T 淋巴细胞，体积和比重较其他细胞大，可通过速率沉降（rate sedimentation，即体积分离）或平衡沉降（equilibrium sedimentation，即密度分离）将 T 淋巴细胞与 B 淋巴细胞加以分离。

本实验采用 Ficoll 密度梯度离心法分离外周血单个核细胞（peripheral blood mononuclear cell，PBMC）。淋巴细胞分离液（Ficoll，聚蔗糖—泛影葡胺）比重为 1.077±0.001，是介于 1.075 与 1.092 之间的等渗密度梯度液。离心后，红细胞最重，沉至管底；多形核白细胞比重在 1.092 左右，沉于红细胞之上、分层液之下；淋巴细胞和单核细胞的比重小于或等于分层液比重，离心后漂浮于分层液的液面上，也可有少部分细胞悬浮在分层液中。吸取分层液液面的细胞，就可从外周血中分离到单个核细胞。

**【实验器材】**

（1）比重为 1.077±0.001 的聚蔗糖—泛影葡胺（商品名为淋巴细胞分离液）、pH7.4 的 Hank's 液（无 $Ca^{2+}$、$Mg^{2+}$）、含 10%胎牛血清的 RPMI-1640 溶液、0.2%台酚蓝染色

# VI. E-Rosette Forming Cell Test

**【Aim】**

Get familiar with the principle, procedure and usage of E-rosette forming cell test.

**【Principle】**

Normal T lymphocytes in human peripheral blood has E-receptor (CD2), which can combine with glycoprotein on the membrane of sheep red blood cells and it is a unique surface marker of human T lymphocytes. E-receptor can combine with animal red blood cells in vitro, for example, sheep red blood cells, forming E-rosette in which T lymphocyte is the center and surrounded by red blood cells. It has been proved that more than 90% T lymphocytes and some mononuclear macrophages have E-receptors. Once T lymphocytes and sheep red blood cells are mixed together, sheep red blood cells will attach to T lymphocytes and rosette will be formed. The method of detecting T lymphocyte through rosette forming is called E-rosette forming test. The test can be used to quantitate T lymphocytes, therefore can help us to evaluate the cellular immune state, the prognosis of certain diseases, and the efficacy of drugs.

The test is helpful to identify and quantitate T lymphocytes in human peripheral blood. Meanwhile, the size of T lymphocytes bound with SRBC is bigger than other cells, so we can separate T lymphocytes from B lymphocytes with rate sedimentation or equilibrium sedimentation.

In this test, we separate peripheral blood mononuclear cells by Ficoll-Urografin density gradient centrifugation. The specific gravity of lymphocyte separation medium(LSM) is 1.077±0.001, and it is an isotonic density gradient between 1.075 and 1.092. Diluted blood is layered after centrifugation. Red blood cells are the heaviest and sedimented to the bottom of the tube. Polymorphonuclear leukocytes are above red blood cells and beneath LSM since their density is about 1.092. Mononuclear cells and lymphocytes exist in the interface of LSM, and some are mixed in it; because their specific gravity is smaller than or equal to that of LSM. Peripheral blood mononuclear cells are collected from the interface of LSM.

**【Materials and Equipment】**

(1) Ficoll-Urografin which specific gravity is 1.077±0.001 (trade name is lymphocyte separation medium, LSM), pH7.4 Hank's solution (without $Ca^{2+}$, $Mg^{2+}$), RPMI-1640 containing 10% FCS(fetal calf serum), 0.2% trypan blue staining fluid (prepare with normal

液（用生理盐水或等渗的 PBS 配制）、肝素（用 Hank’s 液或生理盐水稀释成 500U/mL）、0.5% SRBC 悬液。

(2) 毛细滴管、1mL 和 10mL 刻度吸管、注射器、碘酒、75%酒精、无菌棉球、止血带、血球计数板、普通光学显微镜。

(3) 离心机、尖吸管、载玻片、瑞氏染液等。

【实验方法】

(1) 在试管中加入适量淋巴细胞分离液。

(2) 取肝素抗凝静脉血与等量 Hank’s 液或 RPMI-1640 溶液充分混匀，用滴管沿管壁缓慢地将抗凝血混合液叠加于分层液面上，注意保持清楚的界面。2 000r/min 离心 20min。

(3) 离心后管内分为 4 层，上层为血浆和 Hank’s 液，第二层是以单个核细胞为主的白色云雾层狭窄带，还含有血小板，第三层为淋巴细胞分离液，第四层为红细胞。

(4) 将毛细滴管插入云雾层，吸取单个核细胞。置入另一短中试管中，加入 5 倍以上体积的 Hank’s 液或 RPMI-1640 溶液，1 500r/min 离心 10min，共洗涤细胞两次。

(5) 最后一次离心后，弃上清液，加入含有 10%胎牛血清的 RPMI-1640 溶液 1mL，重悬细胞，混匀。取一滴细胞悬液与一滴 0.2%台酚蓝染色液混合，置于血球计数板上，计算四个大方格内的细胞总数，检测单个核细胞浓度和细胞活力。

(6) 用 Hank’s 液将 PBMC 配制成 $10^7$/mL 细胞悬液。

(7) 取 0.1mL 细胞悬液，加入 0.1mL 经 SRBC 吸收的灭活胎牛血清，再加入 0.2mL 0.5% SRBC 悬液，混匀，放入 37℃温箱 5min，500r/min 低速离心 5min，然后放入 4℃冰箱 2h 或过夜。

(8) 取出试管，轻轻使沉淀的细胞悬浮，用尖吸管取出一滴置于载玻片上，涂片，自然干燥，瑞氏染色（加染液 1 滴，染 1min，加蒸馏水 5~6 滴，置 6min，蒸馏水冲洗），吸水纸吸干后镜检，观察花环形成。

【实验结果】

(1) T 淋巴细胞被染成紫蓝色，SRBC 被染成红色。凡个体淋巴细胞表面黏附三个或三个以上 SRBC 为一个花环形成细胞。

(2) 镜下计数 200 个淋巴细胞，求出活性 E-花环形成百分率。

(3) 活性 E-花环形成百分率=E-花环形成细胞数/淋巴细胞总数×100%。

正常参考值：(65.6±8.2) %。

saline or isotonic PBS), heparin (dilute to 500 U/mL with Hank's solution or normal saline), 0.5% SRBC suspension.

(2) Capillary burette, 1mL and 10mL scale straws, syringe, iodine, 75% alcohol, sterile cotton balls, tourniquet, blood counting chamber, ordinary optical microscope.

(3) Centrifuge, pipettes, slides, Wright's stain, etc.

**【Procedures】**

(1) Transfer proper amount of LSM to a tube.

(2) Mix heparinized blood and the equal volume of Hank's solution or RPMI-1640. Carefully overlay the mixed blood with capillary burette over LSM in the tube, maintaining a clear interface. Centrifuge at the speed of 2,000 r/min for 20 minutes.

(3) After centrifugation, the mixture is divided into 4 layers, the top layer is plasma and Hank's solution, the second layer is a layer of white cloudy narrow band mainly containing mononuclear cells, also with platelet, the third layer is LSM, and the fourth layer is red blood cells.

(4) Collect mononuclear cells in the second layer with capillary burette and transfer it to a tube. Add 5 times above volume of Hank's solution or RPMI-1640 in the tube and centrifuge at the speed of 1,500r/min for 10 minutes, wash it twice.

(5) After the last centrifugation, discard the supernatant, add 1mL RPMI-1640 containing 10% FCS, and mix thoroughly. Transfer one drop of 0.2% trypan blue staining fluid and one drop of cell suspension into a tube, mix thoroughly. Drop one drop of the mixture on blood counting chamber, and count the cells in the 4 large squares. Assess the concentration and vitality of the mononuclear cells.

(6) Dilute the cell suspension with Hank's solution, the concentration is expected to be $10^7$/mL.

(7) Transfer 0.1mL cell suspension into a tube, add 0.1mL inactivated FCS absorbed by SRBC and 0.2mL 0.5% SRBC suspension, mix thoroughly, incubate in 37℃ thermostat for 5min, centrifuge at the speed of 500r/min for 5min, and then lay it in 4℃ refrigerator for 2h or overnight.

(8) Take out the tube, make the sedimentary cells resuspend gently, add one drop onto the slide, smear, and dry in the air, dye with Wright's stain (add one drop of staining fluid upon the slide, and dye 1min, add 5-6 drops of distilled water, stand for 6min, rinse with distilled water), absorb water with blotting paper, check the formation of E-rosette under microscope.

**【Results】**

(1) T lymphocytes are stained in purple blue, sheep red blood cells are stained in red. One lymphocyte attached by three or more sheep red blood cells represents one E-rosette forming cell.

(2) 200 lymphocytes are counted each time. Calculate the percentage of vital E-rosette forming.

(3) Percentage of vital E-rosette forming=number of E-rosette forming cells/total number

**【注意事项】**

(1) 最好用新鲜的 SRBC，一般采血后保存于 Alsever 液中，两周内可用。超过两周，与淋巴细胞结合的能力下降。

(2) 从采血到测定不要超过 4h，分离的淋巴细胞放置时间也不要超过 4h，否则 SRBC 受体会自行脱落。可用台酚蓝检查淋巴细胞的活力，活细胞数应不少于 95%。

(3) 计数 E-花环前，应将沉于管底的细胞予以重悬，重悬和混匀细胞要轻柔，只宜轻缓旋转试管，使细胞团块松开即可，不能强力吹打，否则花环会散开消失。

(4) 配制 PBMC 悬液应用 10%~20%胎牛血清为好。不加胎牛血清，E-花环形成率会降低。

of lymphocytes×100%.

Normal reference value: (65.6±8.2)%.

**【Attentions】**

(1) Fresh SRBC is needed which is stored in Alsever solution and used within 2 weeks after collection. Its ability of binding lymphocytes declines over 2 weeks.

(2) The time from collection to detection should be within 4h, and the isolated lymphocytes should not be layed for more than 4h, or SRBC receptor may drop down. The vitality of lymphocytes can be detected with trypan blue staining fluid and the percentage of vital cells must not be lower than 95%.

(3) Resuspend the sedimentary cells gently before check the formation of E-rosette. Be gentle to resuspend, mix, and rotate the tube. Strong percussion should be avoided, or the rosette may disappear.

(4) It is better to prepare PBMC suspension with 10%-20% FCS: Without FCS, the percentage of formation of E-rosette will decline.

# 实验七　T 淋巴细胞转化实验

**【实验目的】**

熟悉 T 淋巴细胞转化实验的原理及方法。

**【实验原理】**

T 淋巴细胞表面有 PHA 受体，T 淋巴细胞在体外培养时，当受到非特异性的促有丝分裂素 PHA 的刺激后，T 淋巴细胞表面的 PHA 受体与 PHA 结合，进行有丝分裂，可转化为淋巴母细胞，细胞的形态和结构发生明显的改变，通过染色镜检，即可计算出淋巴细胞的转化率（图 8）。

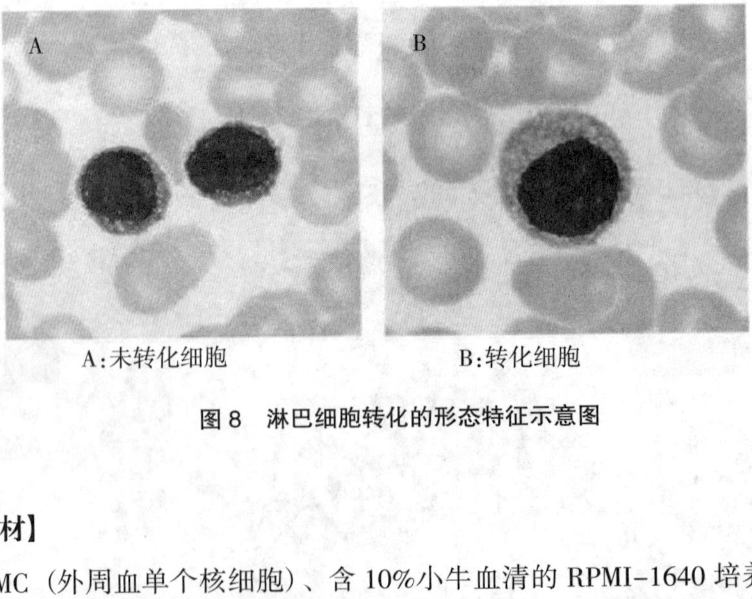


A:未转化细胞　　B:转化细胞

**图 8　淋巴细胞转化的形态特征示意图**

**【实验器材】**

（1）PBMC（外周血单个核细胞）、含 10%小牛血清的 RPMI-1640 培养液、植物血凝素（PHA）（用 RPMI-1640 液配成 1mg/mL，分装小瓶，冷冻保存）。

（2）无菌尖吸管和刻度吸量管、96 孔平底培养板、血球计数板、试管。

（3）$CO_2$ 培养箱、显微镜。

# VII. T Lymphocyte Transformation Test

**【Aim】**

Get familiar with the principle and procedure of T lymphocyte transformation test.

**【Principle】**

T lymphocyte has PHA receptor on its surface, which can interact with PHA, a nonspecific mitogenic hormone and be activated. T lymphocytes in vitro will mitose and transform into lymphoblasts with the morphology and structure changed. Stain and observe under microscope, we can calculate the percentage of the transformed lymphocytes (Figure 8).

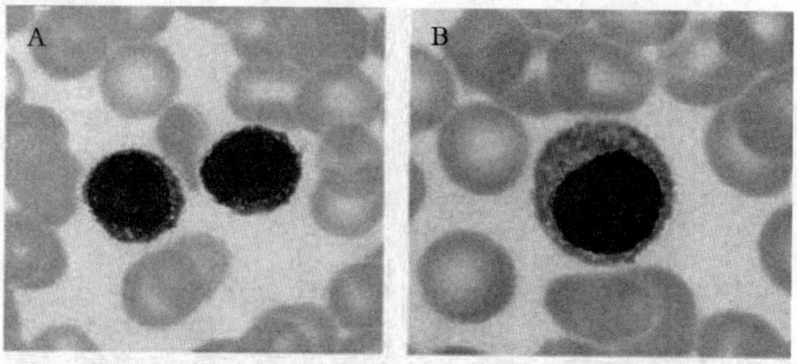


A: untransformed cell B: transformed cell

Figure 8 The Morphological Characteristics of Lymphocyte Transformation

**【Materials and Equipment】**

(1) PBMC (peripheral blood mononuclear cell), RPMI-1640 containing 10% FCS, phytohemagglutinin (PHA)(1mg/mL, prepared with RPMI-1640, aliquot into small bottles, cryopreservation).

(2) Sterile pipettes and graduated pipette, 96-well flat-bottomed culture plates, blood counting chamber, tubes.

(3) $CO_2$ incubator, microscope.

**【Procedures】**

(1) Separate PBMC from heparinized blood and adjust to (1-2) $\times10^6$/mL with RPMI-1640 containing 10% FCS after wash. Add PHA to make the final concentration 2μg/mL, and leave a negative control well without adding PHA.

【实验方法】

(1) （无菌操作）从肝素抗凝血中分离外周血单个核细胞，洗涤后用10%小牛血清RPMI-1640调整细胞数为（1~2）$\times10^6$/mL，加入PHA，使最终浓度为2μg/mL，同时做不加PHA的阴性对照孔。

(2) 将上述细胞混合液加入96孔平底培养板中，每孔0.1mL，将培养板放入含有5%$CO_2$的37℃培养箱中培养。

(3) 取上述培养72h后的细胞做涂片，自然干燥，瑞氏染色（加染液1滴，染1min，加蒸馏水5~6滴，置6min，蒸馏水冲洗，吸水纸吸干），镜检。

【实验结果】

按下列公式计算淋巴细胞的转化率：

淋巴细胞的转化率=转化的淋巴细胞数/(转化的淋巴细胞数+未转化的淋巴细胞数）×100%

(2) Transfer 0.1mL above mixture into each well of the 96-well flat-bottomed culture plate and incubate in 37℃ incubator which contains 5%$CO_2$.

(3) Take out the culture plate 72h later. Make smears, dry in air and dye with Wright's stain (place one drop of straining fluid upon the slide, dry 1min, add 5–6 drops of distilled water, stand for 6min, rinse with distilled water, absorb water with blotting paper). Observe under microscope.

**【Results】**

Calculate the percentage of lymphocyte transformation according to the following formula:

Transformation rate of lymphocyte=total number of transformed lymphocytes/ (number of transformed lymphocytes + number of normal lymphocytes) ×100%

# 实验八 免疫标记技术

免疫标记技术是指用荧光素、酶、放射性同位素或电子致密物质等标记抗原或抗体所进行的抗原抗体反应。此技术的优点是特异性强、敏感度高、速度快，既可定性又可定位、定量检测，结果易于观察。常用标记物质有荧光素、酶、放射性同位素（$^{125}I$、$^{32}P$ 等)、生物素、铁蛋白、胶体金和化学发光物质等。

免疫荧光技术（immunofluorescence technique）是最早发展的免疫标记技术，是在免疫学、生物化学和显微镜技术的基础上建立起来的一项技术。免疫荧光技术包括荧光抗体技术（用荧光抗体示踪或检查相应抗原）和荧光抗原技术（用已知的荧光抗原标记物示踪或检查相应抗体），前者较为常用。最常用的荧光素有异硫氰酸荧光素（FITC)、四乙基罗丹明（RB200）和四甲基异硫氰基罗丹明（TRITC）等。在紫外线作用下，荧光素发出荧光，在荧光显微镜下可以直接观察呈现特异荧光的抗原抗体复合物及其存在部位而进行定性和定位；也可与标准品对照得到分析物的浓度而进行定量。荧光抗体技术有直接法和间接法两种基本类型。

直接法是用已知荧光素标记抗体测抗原。其优点为：①干扰因素少，结果易于判断；②特异性强，与其他抗原交叉染色较少；③操作步骤少，简便、省时。其缺点有：①敏感性较低；②每检测一种抗原需制备相应的特异性荧光标记抗体；③只能测抗原。

间接法是最常用的荧光抗体技术，是先将待测（或已知）抗体与含已知（或待测）抗原的标本作用，洗去未结合抗体，再加入荧光素标记的二抗，以检测抗体或抗原。其优点为：①敏感性较直接法高；②制备一种荧光素标记的抗 Ig（二抗）即可检测同一物种的针对不同抗原的某一类 Ig（如 IgG)；③既可测抗体，也可测抗原。其缺点为：①有时易出现非特异性荧光；②操作较烦琐、费时。

# VIII. Immunolabelling Technique

Immunolabelling technique is a kind of antigen-antibody reaction during which antigen or antibody is marked by fluorescein, enzyme, radioisotope or electronic dense substances. This technology has advantages of strong specificity, high sensitivity and fast operation. The result is both qualitative and positioning, quantitative and is easy to be observed. We usually use markers such as fluorescein, enzyme, radioactive isotopes ($^{125}I$, $^{32}P$, etc.), biotin, ferritin, colloidal gold, and chemical luminescence materials.

Immunofluorescence technique is the earliest developed immunolabelling technique which is based on immunology, biochemistry and microscope techniques. Immunofluorescence technique includes fluorescent antibody technique and fluorescent antigen technologies. The former checks unknown antigen with fluorescent antibody and is commonly used. The latter checks unknown antibody with fluorescent antigen. The most commonly used fluorescein is fluorescein isothiocyanate (FITC), tetraethyl rhodamine (RB200) and tetramethyl rhodamine isothio cyanate (TRITC), etc. Fluorescein can send out fluorescence with excitation by UV light and we can observe the antigen-antibody complexes that present special fluorescence under fluorescence microscope directly. We know their quality and position by observing where they exist and can have quantity analysis to know their concentration by comparing with the standard. Fluorescent antibody technique has two basic types: direct method and indirect method.

The direct method detects antigen through tagging antibody by known fluorescein. It has advantages as follows: ①Little interference and easy-judging results; ②Strong specificity and little cross staining with other interfering antigen; ③Few operation steps, simple and time-saving. It also has disadvantages: ①Low sensitivity; ②Need to label the corresponding antibody with special fluorescein during each antigen test; ③It is only for antigen detection.

The most popular method is the indirect fluorescent antibody technology, which is to use known-antibody to react with testing-antigen, or vise versa, and wash away those unbounded antibody. Then we can detect the unknown by adding secondary antibody tagged by fluorescein. Its advantages are as follows: ① Higher sensitivity than direct method. ② The secondary antibodies tagged by fluorescein can be used to detect a class of antibodies against different antigens from the same species(for example, IgG). ③It is both used for antibody and antigen detection. Its disadvantages are below: ①Nonspecific fluorescence shows up easily

## 一、B 淋巴细胞抗原识别受体（SmIg）的检测（直接免疫荧光法）

【实验原理】

SmIg 是 B 淋巴细胞的抗原识别受体，也是 B 淋巴细胞特异性的表面标志，其免疫原性与 Ig 相同，用荧光素标记的抗 Ig 抗体，在适当的条件下可与 SmIg 结合；在荧光显微镜下观察，可见 B 淋巴细胞膜上出现荧光。借以检测 B 淋巴细胞膜上 BCR 的存在。此方法可用来鉴定 B 淋巴细胞。

【实验器材】

(1) 小鼠、异硫氰酸荧光素（FITC）标记的兔抗小鼠 Ig 抗体、pH7.4 Hank’s 液（含 0.1% $NaN_3$）。

(2) 100 目不锈钢网、台式离心机、离心管、试管、玻片、吸管及移液管、玻璃平皿。

(3) 4℃冰箱、荧光显微镜。

【实验方法】

(1) 采用颈椎脱臼法处死小鼠，解剖取出脾脏，置于 100 目不锈钢网上，放入盛有 6mL Hank’s 液的平皿中研磨，混匀。制备浓度为 $1\times10^7$/mL 的细胞悬液。另取一支试管，吸取 $1\times10^7$/mL 的细胞悬液 0.4mL，加 Hank’s 液 3.6mL，即为 $1\times10^6$/mL 的细胞悬液。

(2) 取两支 2mL 离心管，各加入 $1\times10^6$/mL 的细胞悬液 1mL，2 000r/min 离心 3min，弃上清液。一支加入荧光素标记的兔抗小鼠 Ig 抗体 100μL，另一支不加抗体作对照，置于 4℃冰箱内 30min。

(3) 取出离心管，用 Hank’s 液洗涤细胞两次，以去除游离的抗体上清液，最后一次离心后弃上清液，留少许回流液，混匀，滴片，用荧光显微镜观察。

【实验结果】

免疫荧光染色细胞的形态和类型：凡细胞呈现较强黄绿色荧光，有明显的细胞轮廓，并可见环状或两个以上斑点或在细胞的一侧见有帽状结构的为 SmIg 阳性细胞（B 淋巴细胞）；凡呈现微弱、均匀一致的暗淡荧光者为非 B 淋巴细胞。

用钨丝灯光源透射光照明，计算同一视野内的淋巴细胞总数，共计数 200~300 个淋巴细胞，算出其中 SmIg 阳性细胞所占的百分比。

B 淋巴细胞百分比（%）=SmIg 阳性细胞数 / 淋巴细胞总数×100%。

sometimes. ②The operation is tedious and time-consuming.

## ⅰ. Detection of B Lymphocyte Antigen Recognition Receptors (SmIg) (Direct Immunofluorescence Method)

**【Principle】**

SmIg is both antigen recognition receptor and special surface marker of B lymphocytes. It has the same immunogenicity as Ig (immune globulin) and can combine with anti-Ig antibody tagged by fluorescein under appropriate conditions. Fluorescence can be observed on the cytomembrane of B lymphocyte under the fluorescence microscope, which can be used to detect existing of BCR on the cytomembrane of B lymphocyte. This method can be applied to identify B lymphocytes.

**【Materials and Equipment】**

(1) Mouse, rabbit anti-mouse immune globulin antibodies tagged by fluorescein isothiocyanate, pH7. 4 Hank's solution (containing 0.1%$NaN_3$) .

(2) 100-mesh stainless steel wire mesh, desk centrifuge, centrifuge tubes, tubes, slides, straws and pipettes, glass plates.

(3) Refrigerator in 4℃ and fluorescence microscope.

**【Procedures】**

(1) Kill the mouse by cervical dislocation, dissect and take out the spleen on 100 mesh stainless steel wire mesh, grind the spleen in a plate with 6mL Hank's solution. Make spleenocyte suspension with concentration of $1\times10^7$/mL. Suck 0.4mL cell suspension into another tube, add 3. 6mL Hank's solution to obtain $1\times10^6$/mL cell suspension.

(2) Take 2mL-centrifuge tubes, add 1mL $1\times10^6$/mL cell suspension in each tube. Centrifuge them at the speed of 2,000r/min for 3min to discard the supernatant. Add 100μL rabbit anti-mouse immune globulin antibodies tagged by fluorescein isothiocyanate in one tube, and the other one with no antibody as negative control. Put both tubes in 4℃ refrigerator for 30min.

(4) Take out the centrifuge tubes and clear the free antibody in the supernatant of the tubes by washing those cells twice with Hank's solution. Abandon the supernatant after the last centrifuge. Keep a few back-flow and mix them thoronghly. Observe it with fluorescence microscope.

**【Results】**

Morphology and type of cells stained by immunofluorescence: SmIg positive cells ( B lymphocytes) present strong yellow-green fluorescence and have obvious contours. Rings or more than two spots or hat-shaped structure in one side of the cells can be seen. The cells that present uniform faint fluorescence are non-B-lymphocytes.

Count a total number of 200-300 lymphocytes in the same field of vision with the transmission light of tungsten light to calculate the percentage of SmIg positive cells.

Percentage of B lymphocytes (%) = number of SmIg positive cells / number of all lymphocytes × 100%

## 二、酶联免疫吸附实验（ELISA）

【实验目的】

(1) 掌握酶联免疫吸附实验的原理和间接法的实验方法。

(2) 了解抗原竞争法、双抗体夹心法的实验原理及实验方法。

【实验原理】

酶联免疫吸附实验（enzyme-linked immunosorbent assay，ELISA）的基本原理是：由于抗原、抗体的反应在一种固相载体——聚苯乙烯微量滴定板的孔中进行，每加入一种试剂孵育后，可通过洗涤除去游离的反应物，从而保证实验结果的特异性与稳定性，且最后结合在固相载体上的酶量与标本中受检物质的量成一定的比例。加入酶反应的底物后，底物被酶催化变为有色产物，产物的量与标本中受检物质的量直接相关，故可根据颜色的深浅进行定性或定量分析。酶的催化效率很高，从而使该测定方法具有高敏感度。具体的方法较多，有用于检测抗体的间接法、用于检测抗原的双抗体夹心法以及用于检测小分子抗原或半抗原的抗原竞争法等。比较常用的是 ELISA 双抗体夹心法及 ELISA 间接法。酶联免疫吸附实验的特点是敏感性高、特异性强、操作简易、结果容易观察，经常应用于经免疫酶染色的各种细胞内成分的定位、研究抗酶抗体的合成、显现微量的免疫沉淀反应、定量检测体液中抗原或抗体的成分等方面。

【实验器材】

(1) 包被缓冲液（pH9.6 的 0.05mol/L 碳酸盐缓冲液）、洗涤缓冲液（pH7.4 的 0.15mol/L PBS）、底物缓冲液（pH5.0 柠檬酸-磷酸氢二钠）、终止液（2mol/L 的 $H_2SO_4$）、抗原、抗体及酶标记抗体、正常人血清和阳性对照血清、TMB。

(2) 聚苯乙烯板（简称酶标板）40 孔或 96 孔、ELISA 检测仪、50μL 和 60μL 微量加样器、塑料滴头、小毛巾、洗涤瓶、小烧杯、玻璃棒、试管、吸管、量筒等。

(3) 4℃冰箱、37℃温箱。

【实验方法】

1. ELISA 间接法

ELISA 间接法是检测抗体最常用的方法，其原理为：利用酶标记的抗抗体检测已与固相结合的受检抗体，故称为间接法。

(1) 包被固相抗原：用包被缓冲液将已知抗原稀释至 1~10μg/mL，在每个聚苯乙烯板的反应孔中加 0.1mL，置于 4℃冰箱中过夜。次日弃去孔内溶液，用洗涤缓冲液洗 3 次，每次 3min，除去未结合的抗原及杂质。

## ii. Enzyme-Linked Immunosorbent Assay (ELISA)

**【Aim】**

(1) To master the principle of enzyme-linked immunosorbent assay (ELISA) and the indirect experimental method.

(2) To know experimental principles and methods of antigen competition and double antibody sandwich method.

**【Principle】**

The basic principle of ELISA is as follows: When assaying antibodies or antigens, it is very convenient to have the antigen and antibody react in the wells of a solid phase carrier—polystyrene microtiter plate. The specificity and stability of the experimental results can be ensured by washing to remove free reactants after addition of a reagent and incubation each time, finally the amount of the enzyme combined on the solid phase carrier is proportional to the amount of substance being tested in the sample. The substrate becomes colored product after catalyzed by enzyme when it is added into the reaction system, and its amount shows direct relationship with the amount of unknown sample. So according to the density of the color we can do qualitative or quantitative analysis. This method has a high sensitivity because of the high efficiency of enzymatic catalysis. There are many specific methods, such as indirect method for detecting antibodies, double antibody sandwich method for detecting antigen, and antigen competition method for detection of small molecular antigen or hapten, etc. Double antibody sandwich method and indirect method of ELISA are commonly used. Because of its characteristics of high sensitivity, strong specificity, easy to operate and observe the results, ELISA is often applied to locate a variety of ingredients in the cell dyed by immune enzyme, to research synthesis of antibodies resistant to enzyme, to show microcrystalline immune precipitation reaction, and to detect those antigens or antibodies in body fluids quantitatively, etc.

**【Materials and Equipment】**

(1) Coating buffer (pH9.6, 0.05mol/L carbonate buffer), washing buffer (pH7.4, 0.15mol/L PBS), substrate buffer (pH5.0 citric acid-disodium hydrogen phosphate), stop buffer(2mol/L $H_2SO_4$), antigen, antibody and enzyme-labelled antibody(ELA), normal human serum and positive control serum, TMB.

(2) Polystyrene board (referred to as ELISA plate) with 40 or 96 wells, ELISA detector, 50μL and 60μL micropipettes, plastic tops, towelette, washing bottles, small beaker, glass rod, tube, straws, measuring cylinder, etc.

(3) 4℃ refrigerator, 37℃ thermostat.

**【Procedures】**

### 1. Indirect ELISA method

Indirect ELISA method uses anti-antibody labeled by enzyme to detect testing antibody bound on solid phase carrier, which is the most commonly used method for antibody detection.

(1) Coat solid phase antigen: Dilute the known antigens to 1 –10μg/mL with coating

(2) 加待检标本：加一定稀释度的待检样品（未知抗体）0.1mL 于上述已包被的反应孔中，置于 37℃温箱中孵育 1h，用洗涤缓冲液洗 3 次，每次 3min，除去未结合的抗体及杂质。同时做空白孔、阴性对照孔及阳性对照孔。

(3) 加酶标抗抗体：于反应孔中加入新鲜稀释的酶标抗抗体（羊抗人 IgG 抗体、鼠抗人 IgG 抗体等抗抗体）0.1mL，置于 37℃温箱中孵育 30~60min，用洗涤缓冲液洗 3 次，每次 3min。

(4) 加底物缓冲液显色：于各反应孔中加入临时配制的 TMB 底物缓冲液 0.1mL，置于 37℃温箱中孵育 10~30min。

(5) 终止反应：于各反应孔中加入终止液 0.05mL。

(6) 判定结果：直接用肉眼观察结果或在 ELISA 检测仪上测各孔的 OD 值。

本法只要更换不同的固相抗原，可以用一种酶标抗抗体检测各种与抗原相应的抗体（图 9）。

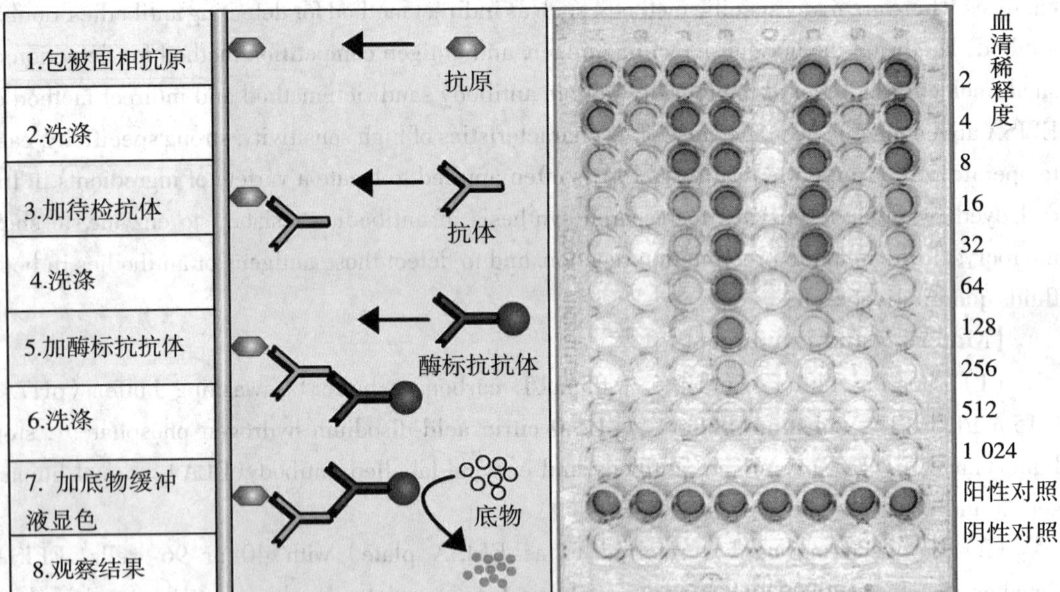


图 9 酶联免疫吸附实验（ELISA）

2. ELISA 双抗体夹心法

ELISA 双抗体夹心法是检测抗原最常用的方法，操作步骤如下：

(1) 包被固相抗体：用 0.05mol/L pH9.0 碳酸盐缓冲液将抗体稀释至蛋白质含量为 1~10μg/mL。在每个聚苯乙烯板的反应孔中加入 0.1mL 稀释的抗体，置于 4℃冰箱中过

buffer, add 0.1mL to each reaction well of polystyrene board and keep them in 4℃ refrigerator through the night. Discard the solution in the well the next day, then wash it 3 times with washing buffer, 3min each time to remove uncombined antigen and impurities.

(2) Add being tested sample: Add 0.1mL being tested sample (unknown antibody) with certain degree of dilution in the coated reaction wells above, incubate in 37℃ thermostat for 1h, wash with washing buffer 3 times, 3min each time to remove uncombined antibodies and impurities. At the same time, make blank well, negative well and positive well as controls.

(3) Add anti-antibody labelled by enzyme: Add 0.1mL fresh diluted anti-antibody labelled by enzyme in the reaction well (sheep anti-human IgG antibody, mouse anti-human IgG antibody, etc. ), incubate in 37℃ thermostat for 30 to 60 minutes. Wash with washing buffer 3 times, 3min each time.

(4) Add substrate buffer to color: Add 0.1mL freshly prepared TMB substrate buffer in each reaction well, incubate in 37℃ thermostat for 10–30min.

(5) The termination reaction: Add 0. 05mL 2mol/L stop buffer in each reaction well.

(6) Observe the result: Observe the result with naked eyes directly or measure OD value of each well on ELISA detector.

By only replacing antigen in solid phase, we can use one anti-antibody labelled by enzyme to detect many antibodies corresponding to its antigen(Figure 9).

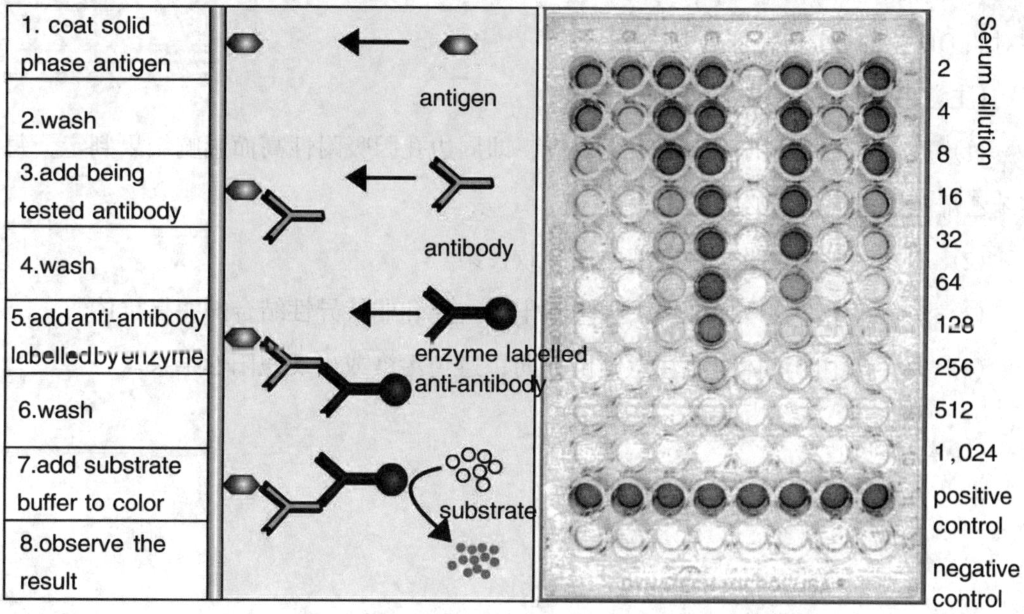


Figure 9 Enzyme-Linked Immunosorbent Assay (ELISA)

## 2. Double antibody sandwich method of ELISA

Double antibody sandwich method of ELISA is the most commonly used method to detect antigen whose operation steps are as follows:

(1) Coat solid phase antibody: Dilute antibodies to 1–10μg/mL of protein content with

夜。次日，弃去孔内溶液，用洗涤缓冲液洗 3 次，每次 3min，除去未结合的抗体及杂质。

(2) 加待检标本：加一定稀释度的待检样品 0.1mL 于上述已包被之反应孔中，置于 37℃温箱中孵育 1h。然后用洗涤缓冲液洗 3 次，每次 3min，除去未结合的抗原及杂质。同时做空白孔、阴性对照孔及阳性对照孔。

(3) 加酶标抗体：于各反应孔中加入新鲜稀释的酶标抗体 0.1mL，置于 37℃温箱中孵育 0.5~1h，用洗涤缓冲液洗 3 次，每次 3min，除去未结合的酶标抗体。

(4) 加底物缓冲液显色：于各反应孔中加入临时配制的 TMB 底物缓冲液 0.1mL，置于 37℃温箱中孵育 10~30min。

(5) 终止反应：于各反应孔中加入终止液 0.05mL。

(6) 判定结果：直接用肉眼观察结果或在 ELISA 检测仪上测各孔的 OD 值。

根据同样原理，可用双抗原夹心法测定标本中的抗体。

【实验结果】

可于白色背景上，直接用肉眼观察结果。反应孔内颜色越深，阳性程度越强，阴性反应为无色或极浅，依据所呈颜色的深浅，以“+”“-”号表示。也可测 OD 值：在 ELISA 检测仪上，于 450nm 处，以空白对照孔调零后测各孔的 OD 值，若大于规定的阴性对照 OD 值的 2.1 倍，即为阳性。

【注意事项】

(1) 聚苯乙烯板有时可出现边缘效应，即周边孔因吸附性高而影响结果判定，每批聚苯乙烯板购进后应做必要的抽查。

(2) 加样时要避免吸头碰到液面而导致污染。

(3) 洗板要干净，以保证洗去吸附不牢的抗原和非特异性结合的酶标抗体。

(4) 去除孔中的液体时要注意倾倒方向，避免污染或出现假阳性结果。

0.05mol/L pH9.0 carbonate buffer. Add 0.1mL those diluted antibodies in each well of polystyrene board, keep them in 4℃ refrigerator through the night. Discard the solution in the hole the next day and wash with washing buffer 3 times, 3min each time, to remove uncombined antibodies and impurities.

(2) Add being tested sample: Add 0.1mL being tested sample with certain degree of dilution in the coated reaction wells above, incubate in 37℃ thermostat for 1h, wash it with washing buffer 3 times, 3min each time to remove uncombined antigen and impurities. At the same time, make blank well, negative well and positive well as controls.

(3) Add antibody labelled by enzyme: Add 0.1mL freshly diluted antibody labelled by enzyme in each reaction well, incubate in 37℃ thermostat for 0.5–1h, wash it 3 times with washing buffer, 3min each time to remove uncombined antibodies labelled by enzyme.

(4) Add substrate buffer to color: Add 0.1mL freshly prepared TMB substrate buffer in each reaction well, incubate in 37℃ thermostat for 10–30min.

(5) The termination reaction: Add 0. 05mL 2mol/L stop buffer in each reaction well.

(6) Observe the result: Observe the result with the naked eyes directly or measure OD value of each well on ELISA detector.

In the same way, we can use double antigen sandwich method to detect unknown antibody in samples.

**【Results】**

We can observe the result directly with naked eyes against a white background. In the reaction well, the deeper the color, the stronger the degree of positive reaction, and there is no or very light color in negative reactions. We can use "+" "–"or measure value of OD to describe the extent of the color. Any reacting well whose OD value is greater than 2.1 times of that of the negative well in ELISA detector at 450nm is positive after zeroing with blank control.

**【Attentions】**

(1) Edge effect may appear in polystyrene board sometimes. That is to say, the surrounding wells with high adsorption may affect the results, so it is necessary to do spot test for each batch of purchased polystyrene boards.

(2) Caution to avoid tip touching the surface of samples during adding reagents in case of contamination.

(3) Clean the board to ensure that all the infirm absorbed antigens and non-specific adsorbed enzyme labelled antibodies are washed.

(4) Pay attention to the direction when dumping the liquid in the wells in case of contamination or false positive results.

# 实验九 豚鼠血清过敏反应

实验动物过敏症属于Ⅰ型超敏反应，与临床常见的青霉素和异种动物血清引起的过敏性休克相似，通过实验可进一步加深对Ⅰ型超敏反应机理的理解，提高医护人员对人类过敏性休克重要性的认识。

**【实验目的】**

掌握Ⅰ型超敏反应皮肤实验原理、特点、方法和临床意义；了解Ⅰ型超敏反应皮肤实验方法。

**【实验原理】**

马血清等变应原可引起人和动物的过敏性休克。豚鼠对马血清敏感，极易刺激豚鼠产生 IgE，引发过敏性休克。先给动物注射异种蛋白，经过一定时间后，动物产生的 IgE 抗体结合于肥大细胞和嗜碱性粒细胞上，动物处于致敏状态。当第二次给动物注射较大量相同抗原时，抗原与细胞表面的 IgE 结合，导致肥大细胞和嗜碱性粒细胞脱颗粒，释放活性介质，作用于效应器官，产生严重的过敏性休克。

**【实验器材】**

(1) 豚鼠（250g 左右）、马血清、鸡卵白蛋白。

(2) 无菌盐水、注射器、解剖器具、碘酒、酒精。

**【实验方法】**

(1) 取健康豚鼠两只，其中一只腹腔注射 1:10 稀释的马血清 0.5mL，使其建立致敏状态，另一只不做任何处理或注射 100mg/mL 鸡卵白蛋白盐水溶液 0.5mL 作为对照。

(2) 两周后，给两只豚鼠心脏内注射马血清 1~2mL，注射 1~5min 后观察动物的状态。

(3) 对死亡的豚鼠进行解剖，观察其各脏器的变化。

**【实验结果】**

用马血清致敏的那只豚鼠，数分钟后即兴奋不安、抓鼻、咳嗽、打喷嚏，继而竖

# IX. Anaphylactic Shock in Guinea Pig

Experimental animal allergy belongs to type Ⅰ hypersensitivity reaction, which is similar to the anaphylactic shock caused by penicillin and heterologous animal serum commonly seen in clinics. This experiment expands the understanding of the mechanism of type Ⅰ hypersensitivity reaction, improving the awareness of importance of human anaphylactic shock in medical staff.

**【Aim】**

To master the principle, characteristics, methods and clinical significance of the skin test of type Ⅰ hypersensitivity; to understand the method of the skin test of type Ⅰ hypersensitivity.

**【Principle】**

Horse serum and other allergens can cause anaphylactic shock in humans and animals. Guinea pig is sensitive to horse serum, which can stimulate guinea pig to produce IgE easily, and cause anaphylactic shock. Firstly, inject foreign protein into animals to induce the production of IgE. After a certain period of time, IgE antibodies bind to mast cells and basophils, leading animals to a sensitization state. When animals are injected with a large amount of the same antigen in the second time, antigen would bind with IgE on the surface of cells, resulting in degranulation of mast cells and basophils to release active mediators, which can act on the effector organs and lead to severe anaphylactic shock.

**【Materials and Equipment】**

(1) Guinea pig (about 250g), horse serum, chicken albumin.

(2) Sterile saline solution, syringes, anatomical tools, iodine, alcohol.

**【Procedures】**

(1) Take two healthy guinea pigs. Inject 0.5mL of diluted horse serum (usually 1:10) into the abdominal cavity of one of the guinea pigs, to establish a sensitization state. Inject 0.5mL of the 100mg/mL chicken albumin saline solution into another as a control or give it no treatment.

(2) After two weeks, inject 1–2mL of horse serum into the heart of two guinea pigs. Observe the condition of them in 1–5min.

(3) Dissect the dead guinea pig, then observe the changes of the organs.

**【Results】**

The experimental guinea pig, which is injected with horse serum, is characterized by

毛、呼吸急促，出现痉挛性跳跃、大小便失禁等表现，全身倒向一侧，最终休克死亡。对其进行解剖，可见肺脏极度气肿，充满整个胸腔。另一只对照用豚鼠（仅接受马血清注射一次）则安然无恙，其临床表现与正常豚鼠一样。

**【注意事项】**

心脏注射时必须准确，有回血时再注射，注射过程中不能人为地造成心脏损伤，注射速度不能太快，固定豚鼠要适度，否则易造成窒息，影响观察结果。

anxiety, scratching the nose, coughing, sneezing, ruffling of hair, shortness of breath, spastic jumps, incontinence, the whole body falling to one side, and shock and die. On autopsy, pneumonedema could be found, the lung is characteristically over inflated. The control guinea pig, which is injected with horse serum only once is safe, and its clinical manifestation is the same as that of normal guinea pigs.

**【Attentions】**

Be accurate when injecting into the heart. Inject with the blood back and do not injure the heart artificially. Be slow when injecting. Fix guinea pig moderately or it would be suffocated easily and affect the observation of the result.

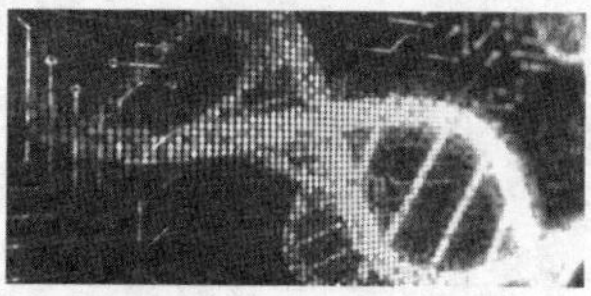

# 第二篇　医学微生物学实验

# Part 2　Medical Microbiology Experiment

# 实验十 细菌的形态与结构

**【实验目的】**

掌握细菌的基本形态与结构特点。

**【实验原理】**

通过本实验认识与熟悉细菌的基本形态与结构特点。各种细菌在一定条件下，均维持一定的形态和结构。细菌的形态与结构是鉴别细菌种类的依据之一，细菌结构又与其致病性强弱、免疫发生机制有一定关系。

**【实验器材】**

(1) 普通光学显微镜、镜油、擦镜纸。

(2) 观察标本：

① 球菌：葡萄球菌、链球菌、淋球菌涂片标本。

② 杆菌：大肠杆菌涂片标本。

③ 弧菌：霍乱弧菌涂片标本。

④ 荚膜：肺炎双球菌荚膜标本。

⑤ 鞭毛：变形杆菌鞭毛标本。

⑥ 芽胞：破伤风梭菌芽胞标本。

**【实验方法与结果】**

(1) 用油镜观察细菌的基本形态，比较其形状、大小、排列及染色性。

(2) 观察细菌特殊结构：荚膜的特点，如大小、颜色及其与菌体的关系；鞭毛的特点，如鞭毛的形态、数目及位置；芽胞的形状、颜色及位置。

(3) 观察标本的同时，在实验报告纸上画出细菌基本形态及特殊结构，并用文字描述。

**【思考题】**

(1) 细菌的基本结构包括哪些？

(2) 细菌有哪些特殊结构？各有什么功能？

# X. Morphology and Structure of the Bacteria

**【Aim】**

To master the basic morphology and structural characteristics of bacteria.

**【Principle】**

Get familiar with the basic morphology and structural characteristics of bacteria through this test. Under certain conditions, every kind of bacteria maintains a certain morphology and structure. Identification of bacterial species depends on their form and structure, and the structure of bacteria is related with their pathogenicity and immunogenicity.

**【Materials and Equipment】**

(1) Ordinary optical microscope, immersion oil, lens paper.

(2) Specimens:

① Coccus: Smear samples of *Staphylococcus*, *Streptococcus*, and *Gonococcus*.

② Bacillus: Smear sample of *Escherichia coli*.

③ Vibrio: Smear sample of *Vibrio cholerae*.

④ Capsule: Capsule specimen of *Streptococcus pneumoniae*.

⑤ Flagellum: Flagellum specimen of *Bacillus proteus*.

⑥ Spores: Spore specimen of *Clostridium tetani*.

**【Methods and Results】**

(1) Observe the basic forms of bacteria under oil immersion lens, compare their shapes, sizes, arrangements and staining properties.

(2) Observe the special structure of bacteria: capsular characteristics: the size, color and the relationship with thallus; flagellate characteristics: the shape, number and location; sporal characteristics: the shape, color and location.

(3) Observe the samples and draw up the basic form and the special structure of bacteria at the same time, and describe them appropriately.

**【Questions】**

(1) What are the basic structures of bacteria?

(2) What are the special structures of bacteria and their functions?

# 实验十一 细菌不染色标本观察法

**【实验目的】**

了解细菌不染色标本的观察方法。

**【实验原理】**

许多细菌标本不经染色直接镜检，可观察其在生活状态下的形态及运动情况。有的杆菌、弧菌有鞭毛，有鞭毛的细菌具有动力，常能朝着一定方向移动，用适当的方法可在普通光学显微镜下观察。对于不染色标本，常用悬滴法或压滴法观察细菌的运动。

**【实验器材】**

(1) 菌种：变形杆菌、葡萄球菌 8~12h 培养物。

(2) 凹玻片、盖玻片、凡士林。

(3) 普通光学显微镜。

**【实验方法】**

1.悬滴法

(1) 取洁净凹玻片一张，在凹窝周围涂上凡士林。

(2) 取一环变形杆菌或葡萄球菌培养物，放于干净的盖玻片中央。

(3) 将涂有凡士林的凹玻片反转（凹向下），凹窝对准盖玻片的菌液滴，黏住盖玻片再反转凹玻片，用接种环柄轻压盖玻片周围，使之与凹窝边缘黏紧。

(4) 凹玻片置于镜台上，先在低倍镜下找到细菌悬滴，然后换用高倍镜观察，即可看到在较暗的视野中有反光较强的闪动或流动的菌体。

(5) 观察结果：镜下可见有鞭毛的变形杆菌运动活泼，并可向不同方向迅速运动；无鞭毛的葡萄球菌只在一定范围内作位移不大的颤动。

悬滴法镜检如图 10 所示。

# Ⅺ. Observation of Unstained Bacteria Specimen

**【Aim】**

Get to know the method of observation of unstained bacteria specimen.

**【Principle】**

Many bacteria specimens can be observed directly through microscope for their morphology and movement without staining. Some bacillus and vibrio have flagella, which make the bacteria move toward a certain direction. These movements can be observed under ordinxry optical microscope with proper methods, for example, hanging drop method or pressure drop method, which are commonly used.

**【Materials and Equipment】**

(1) Bacteria: *Bacillus proteus* and *Staphylococcus* cultured for 8–12 hours.

(2) Concave slide, coverslip, vaseline.

(3) Ordinary optical microscope.

**【Methods】**

## 1. Hanging drop method

(1) Take a clean *concave slide*, coat *vaseline around the* concave.

(2) Place a loop of *Bacillus proteus* or *Staphylococcus* culture at the center of a clean coverslip.

(3) Turn over the concave slide, cover on the coverslip and make the concave aim at the bacteria droplets on the coverslip. Press slightly to paste on the coverslip and then reverse them. Slightly press the edge of coverslip with the handle of inoculation loop to make it stick tightly to the edge of the concave.

(4) Place the concave slide on the microscope stage, find the bacterial suepension first under low power lens, then observe under high power lens. Some strong reflective flashing or cell mobility in the dark vision should be seen.

(5) The result of the observation: Flagellated *Bacillus proteus* rapidly move towards different directions; *Staphylococcus* without flagella only vibrate within a certain range.

The hanging drop method is shown in Figure 10.

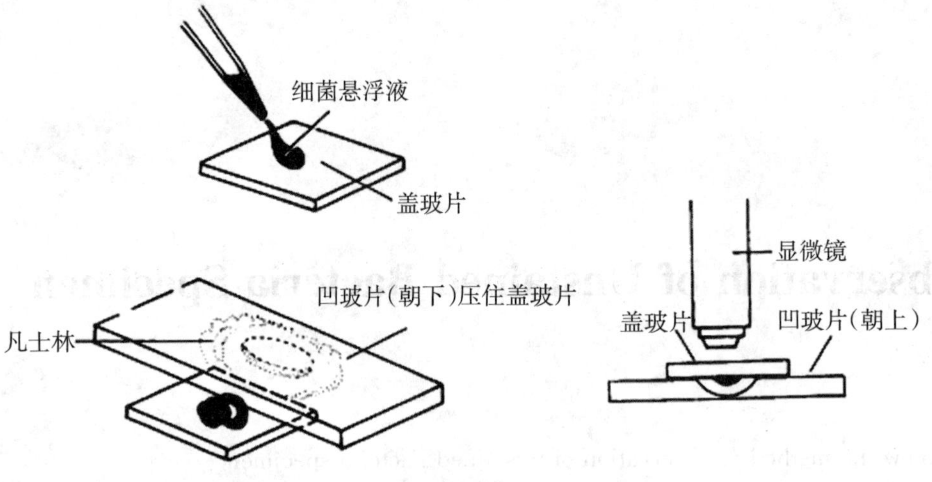


图 10　悬滴法镜检

2. 压滴法

(1) 取洁净载玻片 1 张。

(2) 用接种环取葡萄球菌或变形杆菌液体培养物加于载玻片中央。

(3) 将擦净的盖玻片置于菌液上，覆盖时，先用盖玻片一边接触菌液，缓缓放下盖玻片，防止玻片间产生气泡，滴加菌液量以覆盖玻片后无菌液溢出盖玻片为度。

(4) 将载玻片置于镜台上，用低倍镜找到标本，再换高倍镜观察。

压滴法镜检如图 11 所示。

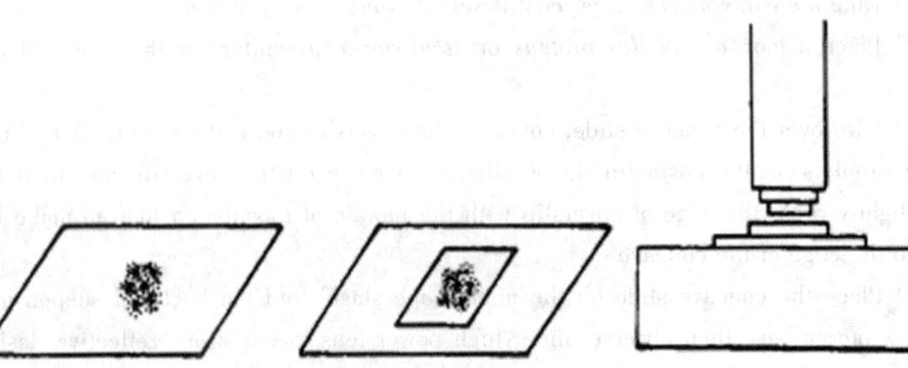

图 11　压滴法镜检

【实验结果】

变形杆菌有明显的定向运动，从一处运动到另一处，即穿梭般运动，这说明其有鞭毛。葡萄球菌只有布朗运动，在原位颤动。

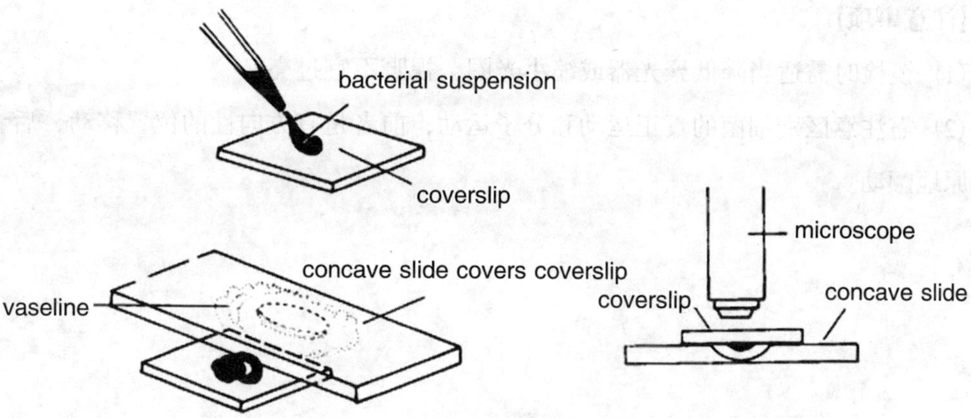


Figure 10 Observation of Hanging Drop Method

2. Pressure drop method

(1) Take a clean slide.

(2) Using an inoculation loop, place the liquid culture of *Staphylococcus* or *Bacillus proteus* at the center of the slide, respectively.

(3) Cover a clean coverslip on the bacterial suspension: Contact the bacterial suspension with a side of the coverslip firstly, and then lay down the coverslip slowly to avoid air bubbles produced between the slides. The amount of bacterial suspension meets the demand that no bacterial suspension overflows when covering the slide.

(4) Place the slide on the microscope stage, find the specimen under low power lens, and then observe it under high power lens.

The pressure drop method is shown in Figure 11.

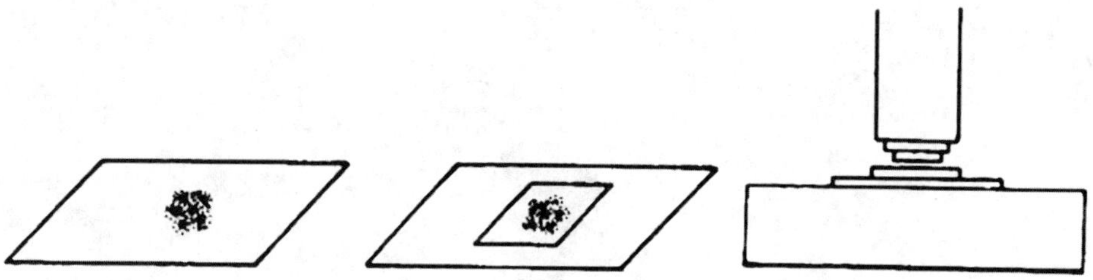

Figure 11 Observation of Pressure Drop Method

**【Results】**

*Bacillus proteus* has a significant directional movement, from one place to another. The shuttle-like movement indicates the presence of flagella. *Staphylococcus* has only Brownian motion, and vibrates in situ.

**【注意事项】**

(1) 镜检时需适当降低聚光器或缩小光圈，视野不宜过亮。

(2) 需注意区别细菌的真正运动和分子运动，前者是有方向性的位置移动，后者则只在原地颤动。

**【Attentions】**

(1) During microscopic examination, reduce the light appropriately to make sure the vision field is not too bright.

(2) Distinguish between the movement of bacteria and molecular motion. The former is directional movement, while the latter is vibration in situ.

# 实验十二 细菌染色标本检查法

细菌个体微小，呈半透明状。未经染色的细菌，在光学显微镜下只能观察到其大致形态和大小。经过染色的细菌，不但能清楚地观察到其各种形态，还可对其进行初步鉴别。

染色方法有单染色与复染色，只用一种染料使细菌着色的方法称为单染色法，可清楚观察细菌的形态、大小，但对细菌无鉴别价值；用两种以上染料染色的方法叫复染色法，对细菌有辅助鉴别意义，主要有革兰（Gram’s）染色法、抗酸染色法。

## 一、革兰染色法

【实验目的】

通过本实验掌握细菌涂片标本的制备法，掌握革兰染色法的原理与方法。

【实验原理】

革兰染色法是一种复染法，是细菌学中最重要的染色方法之一。根据染色的结果将细菌分为革兰阳性菌和革兰阴性菌两大类。革兰阳性菌等电点（pI 2~3）比阴性菌等电点（pI 4~5）低，在相同 pI 条件下，革兰阳性菌所带负电荷比革兰阴性菌多，故与带正电荷的结晶紫染料结合得较牢固；革兰阳性菌细胞内有某种特殊的化学成分，一般认为是核糖核酸镁盐与多糖的复合物，它与染料——媒染剂复合物相结合，使已着色的细菌不易脱色。革兰阳性菌的细胞壁通透性比阴性菌的低，脱色剂（95%酒精）不易通过革兰阳性菌的细胞壁，将碘和染料的复合物溶解洗出，故不易脱色而保留了紫色。革兰阴性菌等电点（pI 4~5）较革兰阳性菌高，菌体含核糖核酸镁盐少，细胞壁结构较疏松，脱色剂易渗入，故易脱去紫色而后染上复红的红色。

【实验器材】

(1) 菌种：大肠杆菌、葡萄球菌 18~24h 固体培养物。

(2) 染液：革兰一液（结晶紫液）、革兰二液（卢戈碘液）、革兰三液（95%酒精）、革兰四液（稀释苯酚复红溶液）。

(3) 普通光学显微镜、载玻片、镜油、接种环、酒精灯等。

# Ⅻ. Observation of Stained Bacteria Specimen

Bacteria are small and semi-translucent. Without staining, only the general shape and size can be observed under the optical microscope. After being stained, the various forms of bacteria can be clearly observed, and it can be used for preliminary identification of bacteria.

The staining methods include simple stain and counter stain. Simple stain uses only one dye to color the bacteria. It clearly shows the bacterial morphology and size, but has no diagnostic value. The staining method using two or more kinds of dyes is called counter stain, which is assisted in identification of bacteria, mainly includes Gram's staining, acid-fast staining, etc.

## ⅰ. Gram's Staining

**【Aim】**

To grasp the preparation of bacterial smears, master the principles and methods of Gram's staining.

**【Principle】**

Gram's staining, a kind of counter stain, is one of the most important bacterial staining methods. According to the results of Gram's staining, bacteria can be divided into Gram-positive bacteria and Gram-negative bacteria. The isoelectric point of Gram-positive bacteria(pI 2–3) is lower than that of Gram-negative one(pI 4–5). At the same pI, Gram-positive bacteria are more negatively charged than Gram-negative bacteria, so the former can bound with positively charged crystal violet dye more firmly. There is a special chemical composition in the cells of Gram-positive bacteria, which is generally considered to be the complex of ribonucleic acid magnesium salt and polysaccharide, and it binds with the dye—mordant complexes. This binding makes the pigmented bacteria difficult to destain. Moreover, the permeability of the cell wall in Gram-positive bacteria is lower than that of Gram-negative bacteria, it is not so easy for decolorizing agent (95% alcohol) to pass through the cell wall of Gram-positive bacteria and to dissolve and washout the complex of iodine and dyestuff, so the bacteria keep the purple color. Gram-negative bacteria's isoelectric point (pI 4–5) is higher than that of Gram-positive bacteria, they contain less ribonucleic acid magnesium salt, and their cell wall structure is loose, so decolorizing agent is easy to penetrate, therefore, purple color is easy to be taken off from Gram-negative bacteria and then they would be stained with fuchsin in red color.

**【实验方法】**

1.制片

取洁净载玻片 1 张，用记号笔将其划分为 3 格，分别挑取葡萄球菌、大肠杆菌斜面培养物少许，在第 1 小格中放置葡萄球菌，第 2 小格中放置大肠杆菌，第 3 小格中放置葡萄球菌和大肠杆菌。在 3 格中分别加 1 滴生理盐水混匀。制作过程如图 12 所示。

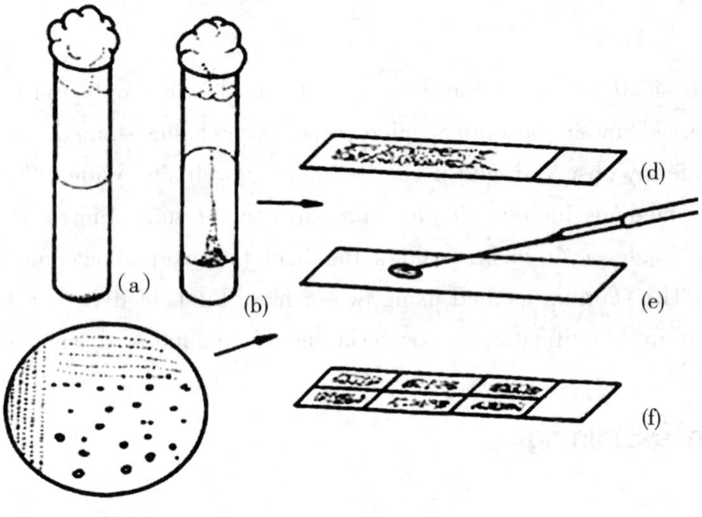


图 12 涂片制作过程

(a) 肉汤增菌液 (b) 半固体斜面 (c) 平板 (d) 菌液涂布 (e) 滴加生理盐水后涂开菌苔或菌落 (f) 多个标本涂片

2.干燥，固定

将上述涂片置于桌面上，在室温下让其自然干燥；或手持载玻片一端，涂有细菌标本的一面朝上，将载玻片在酒精灯火焰外层（最热部分）来回快速通过 3 次，使涂抹的细菌固定于载玻片上。固定时，温度不能太高，以手背皮肤触及载玻片时不感觉过烫为宜。千万不得将载玻片停留于火焰上灼烤，防止细菌烤焦或玻片碎裂。

3.革兰染色

(1) 初染：在已固定好的标本涂片上滴加革兰一液 1~2 滴，染 1min 后，用细水流轻轻冲洗，甩去积水。

(2) 媒染：加革兰二液 1~2 滴，染 1min 后，用细水流冲洗，甩去积水。

(3) 脱色：加革兰三液 2~3 滴，轻轻晃动玻片 3~5s，斜持玻片，使酒精流去，再滴

**【Materials and Equipment】**

(1) Bacteria: Solid cultures of *Escherichia coli*, *Staphylococcus* which are cultured for 18–24h.

(2) Staining solutions: Gram-solution 1 (crystal violet staining solution), Gram-solution 2 (Lugol's iodine), Gram-solution 3 (95% alcohol), Gram-solution 4 (diluted phenol solution).

(3) Ordinary optical microscope, slides, immersion oil, inoculation loop, alcohol lamp, etc.

**【Procedures】**

### 1. Smear

Take a clean slide, mark out three parts with a marker, put a little culture of *Staphylococcus* in part one, and a little culture of *Escherichia coli* in part two. In part three, put some culture of *Staphylococcus* and *Escherichia coli* together. In each part, drip a drop of normal saline and mix respectively. (Figure 12)

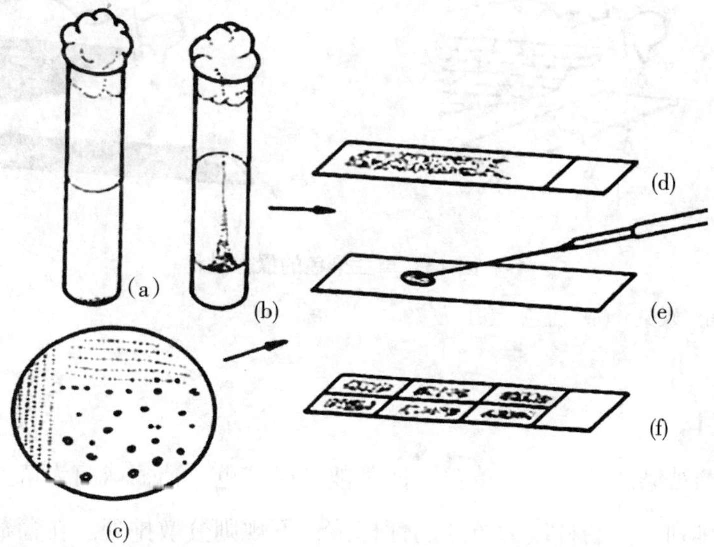


Figure 12 The Production of Smear

(a) enrichment broth (b) semisolid slope (c) flat (d) bacteria coating (e) after dropping normal saline, spread baeteria (f) several smears

### 2. Air dry and fix

Place the above smears on the desk, and let them dry naturally at room temperature, or hold one end of the slide with the coated bacteria specimen side up, make the slide cross through the outer flame layer of alcohol lamp (the hottest part) back and forth quickly for 3 times, so that the bacteria can be fixed on the slide. During fixation, the temperature should not be too high, and the temperature is appropriate when it is touched not too hot on the skin. Do not remain the slide in the flame which could scorch bacteria or cause splintering of slide.

加酒精，如此反复，直到流下的酒精无色或呈淡紫色为止（约 30s），用细水流冲洗，甩去积水。

(4) 复染：加革兰四液 1~2 滴，复染 30s，用细水流冲洗，甩去积水，标本涂片用滤纸吸干，在涂菌处滴加 1 滴香柏油，在油镜下观察。

革兰染色的操作过程如图 13 所示。

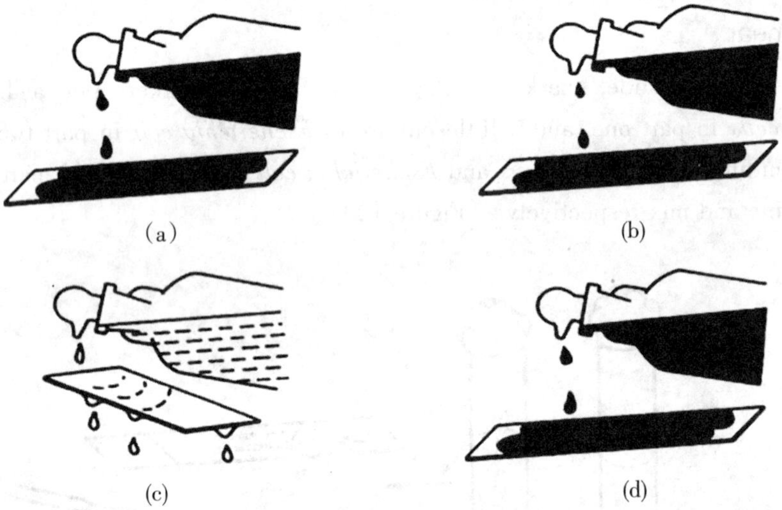

图 13 革兰染色的操作过程

(a) 初染 (b) 媒染 (c) 脱色 (d) 复染

【实验结果】

革兰阳性菌被染成蓝紫色，革兰阴性菌被染成红色。葡萄球菌为革兰阳性球菌，成堆或呈葡萄状排列；大肠杆菌为革兰阴性杆菌，不规则分散排列。在葡萄球菌和大肠杆菌混合涂片中可见被染成蓝紫色的葡萄球菌和被染成红色的大肠杆菌，证明革兰染色可将细菌分为革兰阳性菌和革兰阴性菌。

【注意事项】

(1) 取菌量不可过多，使用生理盐水将菌体研磨成灰白色为宜。涂片太厚或太薄，菌体分散不均匀，都会影响染色结果。固定时应避免菌体过分受热而破坏其形态。

(2) 酒精脱色是革兰染色中的重要环节，如脱色过度，则革兰阳性菌可能被误染为革兰阴性菌；如脱色不够，则革兰阴性菌可能被误染为革兰阳性菌，所以要把握好脱色时间，脱色时间还受涂片厚度的影响。涂片太厚或菌体固定时间过长，都会影响脱色结果。

3. Gram's staining

(1) First staining: Drop 1–2 drops of Grram-solution 1 on the fixed specimen slide and stain for 1min, rinse lightly with slow water, shake off the water.

(2) Mordanting: Add 1–2 drops of Gram-solution 2 and keep for 1min, then wash gently with slow water, shake off the water.

(3) Decoloring: Drop 2–3 drops of Gram-solution 3 and shake the slide gently for 3–5s, hold the slide obliquely to discard the alcohol. Repeat these steps till the alcohol shows colorless or lavender (about 30s). Rinse gently with slow water, shake off the water.

(4) Counter staining: Add 1–2 drops of Gram-solution 4 and stain for 30s, wash with slow water, shake off the water, dry with filter paper. Add 1 drop of cedar oil on the bacterial smear and observe by microscope with oil immersion lens. (Figure 13)

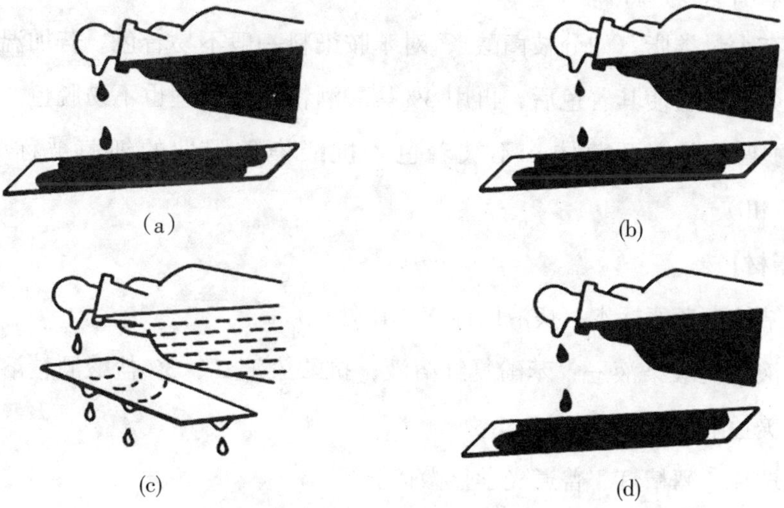


Figure 13 Procedures of Gram's Staining

(a) first staining (b) mordanting (c) decoloring (d) counter staining

**【Results】**

Gram-positive bacteria are dyed in bluish violet, while Gram-negative bacteria are dyed in red. *Staphylococcus* is a kind of Gram-positive cocci, which is in heaps or grape-like arrangement. *Escherichia coli* is Gram-negative bacillus, which is in irregularly dispersed arrangement. In the mixed smear, the bluish violet *Staphylococcus* and red *Escherichia coli* could be seen. The result shows the bacteria can be divided into Gram-positive bacteria and Gram-negative bacteria through Gram's staining.

**【Attentions】**

(1) The amount of bacteria for making smear should not be too much, it is appropriate to grind it into off-white by using normal saline. Smear being too thick or too thin, uneven dispersion of bacteria, will affect the staining results. Avoid excessive heat in fixation, or it will cause damage to the bacteria.

【思考题】

(1) 为什么通过革兰染色细菌得到阳性和阴性两种结果?

(2) 革兰染色有什么应用?

## 二、抗酸染色法

【实验目的】

掌握齐—尼 (Ziehl-Neelsen) 抗酸染色法的原理、操作技术及对染色结果的判读原则。熟悉分枝杆菌的形态。

【实验原理】

分枝杆菌属的细菌具有抗酸性，抗酸染色法是一种鉴别分枝杆菌的方法。分枝杆菌属的细菌，如结核分枝杆菌 (*Mycobacterium tuberculosis*) 和麻风分枝杆菌 (*M. leprae*)，细胞壁中含有大量类脂 (如分枝菌酸)，对苯胺染料一般不易着色。若加温、延长染色时间或提高染液浓度使其着色后，再用 3%盐酸酒精溶液处理也不易脱色。而非抗酸性菌细胞内的染料易离开菌体，不被着色。抗酸染色阳性的细菌被称为抗酸杆菌 (acid-fast bacilli)。

【实验器材】

(1) 肺结核患者痰标本 (痰液已经 NaOH 处理)。

(2) 染液：抗酸染液一：苯酚复红溶液；抗酸染液二：3%盐酸酒精溶液；抗酸染液三：碱性美兰溶液。

(3) 载玻片、酒精灯、普通光学显微镜。

【实验方法】

1.制片

用接种环多次取痰液置于载玻片中央，均匀涂成 1.5cm×2.0cm 的卵圆形厚膜涂片，自然干燥，火焰固定。

2.染色

(1) 在涂面上滴加抗酸染液一 1~2 滴，夹住玻片，置于火焰上缓缓加热，至有蒸汽冒出，约维持 5min (切勿煮沸或煮干，随时补加染液，以防烤干)。冷却后水洗。

(2) 加抗酸染液二 1~2 滴，脱色 30~60s，脱色时轻轻摇动玻片，直至无红色染液流下为止，水洗。

(3) 加抗酸染液三 1~2 滴，复染 60s，水洗，用吸水纸吸干后，用油镜检查。

(2) Decolorization by alcohol is an important step in Gram's staining. Excessive decolorization shall make the Gram-positive bacteria mistakenly be stained as Gram-negative bacteria. But if decolorization is not enough, the Gram-negative bacteria shall be mistakenly stained as Gram-positive bacteria. So the time of decolorization should be contorolled well. The duration of decolorization is affected by the thickness of smears. Thick smears or smears with long time's fixation also affect the staining results.

**【Questions】**

(1) How are positive and negative results obtained in bacterial Gram's staining?

(2) What is the application of Gram's staining?

## ii. Acid-Fast Staining

**【Aim】**

Grasp the principle, technique and interpretation of the results of Ziehl-Neelsen acid-fast staining. Be familiar with the morphology of *Mycobacteria.*

**【Principle】**

*Mycobacterium* has property of acid resistance, and acid-fast staining is a method for its identification. Bacteria of *Mycobacterium,* such as *Mycobacterium tuberculosis* and *Mycobacterium leprae*, their cell walls contain large amounts of lipid (e. g. mycolic acid), which is difficult to be stained by aniline dyes. However, if treat them with heating, prolong the staining time or increase the concentration of the dye, the bacteria can be stained and the stained bacteria are not easy to be decolored when treated by 3% hydrochloric alcohol solution. Dyes in non-acid-fast bacteria are easy to be washed out, therefore the cells are not colored. The bacteria that have positive result in acid-fast staining are called acid-fast bacilli.

**【Materials and Equipment】**

(1) Sputum specimen from tuberculosis patients (pretreated with NaOH).

(2) Staining solution: acid-fast staining solution 1: carbolic fuchsin solution; acid-fast staining solution 2: 3% hydrochloric alcohol solution; acid-fast staining solution 3: alkaline methylene blue solution.

(3) Slides, alcohol lamp, ordinary optical microscope.

**【Procedures】**

### 1. Preparing smear

Pick sterilized sputum repeatedly by inoculation loop, evenly smear to make an oval and thick smear (1.5cm×2.0cm) on the centre of slide, natural drying, fixing through flame.

### 2. Staining

(1) Drop 1–2 drops of acid-fast staining solution 1 on the smear, clamp the slide and place it on the flame to heat slowly. When steam emits, maintain heating for 5min (do not boil or dry it, ready to add more staining solution to prevent being dried). After cooling, wash with water.

(2) Drop 1–2 drops of acid-fast staining solution 2, shaking the slide gently for 30–60s

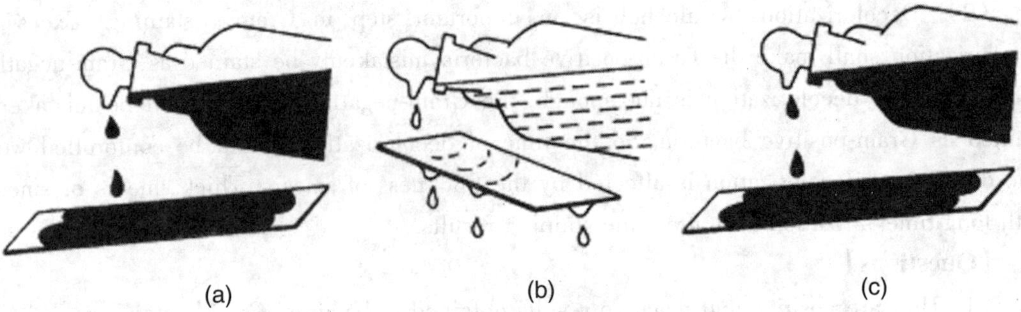


图 14　抗酸染色

(a) 初染 (b) 脱色 (c) 复染

【实验结果】

结核分枝杆菌在淡蓝色的背景下被染成红色，菌体细长或略呈弯曲杆状。非抗酸细菌和涂片中的其他成分均被染成蓝色。

【思考题】

(1) 为什么结核分枝杆菌具有抗酸性?

(2) 抗酸染色过程中应注意什么?

until no red staining solution sheds, and wash.

(3) Drop 1–2 drops of acid-fast staining solution 3, staining for 60s, washing with water, drying with filter paper, observe with oil immersion lens.

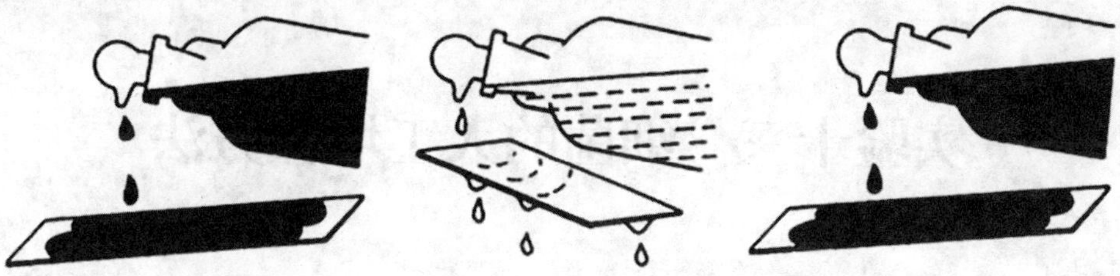

(a) (b) (c)

Figure 14 Acid-Fast Staining

(a) first staining (b) decoloring (c) counter staining

**【Results】**

*Mycobacterium tuberculosis* is dyed into red while the background is in light blue. They are slender or slightly curved rod-shaped bacteria. Non-acid-fast bacteria and other ingredients are dyed into blue.

**【Questions】**

(1) Why the *Mycobacterium tuberculosis* is acid resistant?

(2) What should be paid attention to during the process of acid-fast staining?

# 实验十三 细菌的人工培养方法

## 一、细菌人工培养的接种方法

**【实验目的】**

(1) 掌握平板、斜面、液体和半固体等培养基的接种方法。

(2) 掌握接种环的操作方法，熟悉无菌操作的技术要领。

细菌分离培养法是指将临床材料接种于适当的培养基上进行孵育，分离获得纯种细菌的方法。只有获得纯种细菌才能鉴定细菌，研究细菌的生物学特性、致病性及对药物的敏感性，进而指导临床的疾病治疗。

### (一) 平板划线分离培养法

在自然界中，患者被检材料（痰、便、脓汁及病灶分泌物等）中常有多种细菌混杂在一起，欲证明材料中有无某种细菌存在或专门研究其中某一种细菌时，必须先使各种细菌分散开，方能获得某种单一细菌的培养物，这种技术称为分离培养接种技术。方法有很多，如平板划线法、平板倾注法及动物接种分离法等，前者最为多用。

**【实验原理】**

利用平板划线分离培养法，可分离得到单个菌落，使混杂在一起的细菌分散生长。用黏有混杂菌材料的接种环，在平板培养基表面反复而不重叠地划线，接种环上黏有的细菌逐渐减少，至划线的最后部分细菌可单个留在培养基上，经培养后，生长繁殖成单个菌落。

接种工具有接种环、接种针和玻璃涂布器等。其中，接种环和接种针是最常用的。

(1) 结构：接种环（针）由环（针）、金属柄和绝缘柄三部分组成（如图 15 所示）。环（针）部分一般采用易于传热又不易生锈且经久耐用的铂金丝或镍铬丝制成。接种环的制作过程如图 16 所示。

(2) 使用方法：右手拇指、食指和中指执笔式握执接种环（针），先将环（针）端的金属丝部分置于酒精灯外焰中烧红灭菌，然后使其金属柄部分快速通过火焰两次，以杀灭该段金属表面的微生物，待冷却后即可取标本。用毕，先将接种环（针）端金属丝

# XIII. Artificial Culture of Bacteria

## i. Inoculation Methods for Artificial Culture of Bacteria

**【Aims】**

(1) To master the inoculation methods on plate, slant, liquid and semisolid medium, etc.

(2) To master the ability of using inoculation loop. Be familiar with the key point of aseptic technique.

Bacterial isolation and cultivation is performed in a way that clinical samples are transferred to an appropriate medium to obtain pure culture of bacteria through incubating. It is essential for studying bacterial biological characteristics, pathogenicity and drug sensitivity, then guiding the clinical treatment.

### 1. Streak Plate Method

Samples from patients (such as phlegm, excreta, pus, lesion secretions, etc.) contain multiple bacterial species naturally. To detect or study some special bacteria, you must isolate the bacterial species to get a single colony. It is the so-called isolation and culture technique. It includes the streak plate method, pour plate method, animal inoculation and so on. The streak plate method is the one most often used.

**【Principle】**

Streak plate method can isolate individual colony, making bacterial mixed together grow independently. Rub on the surface of plate medium repeatedly without overlaping by using the inoculation loop where mixed bacteria have stuck on. As the pattern is traced, bacteria are rubbed off the loop onto the medium. The last bacteria be rubbed off the loop should be far enough apart to grow into isolated colonies.

Inoculating devices include inoculation loop, inoculation needle and glass coating machine. Among them, inoculation loop and needle are the most commonly used.

(1) Structure: An inoculation loop (needle) is made up of a small circular ring (needle), a metal holder and an insulated holder (shown in Figure 15). The loop or needle is usually made of nichrome wire or platinum wire, which is with good heat conductivity, stainless and durable. The procedure of making an inoculation loop is shown in Figure 16.

污菌部位稍上部分置于酒精灯外焰中，使热导向环（针），待污菌部位的水分蒸发后，再将接种环（针）灭菌，而后搁于架上，切勿随手乱放，以免灼焦实验台面或其他物品。

(3) 用途：接种环主要用于划线分离、纯种移种及涂片制备等，接种针主要用于穿刺接种细菌及菌落的挑选。

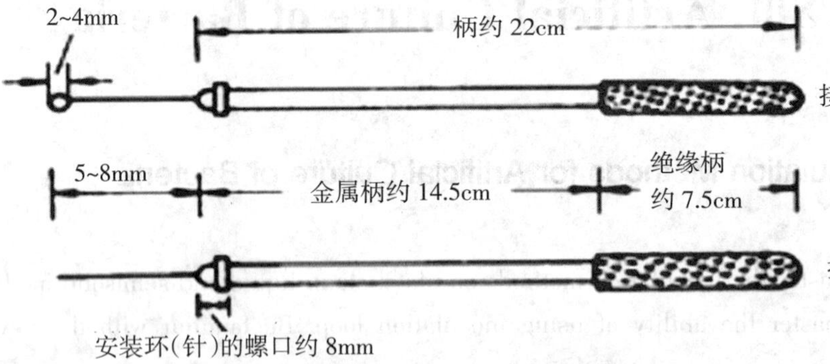


图 15 接种环和接种针示意图

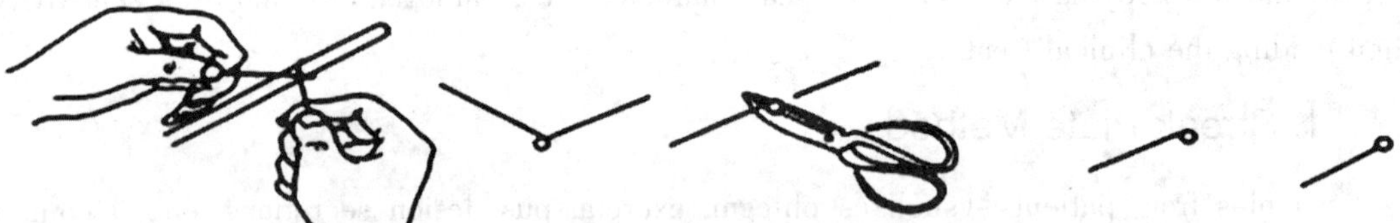

图 16 接种环的制作过程

【实验器材】

(1) 菌种：金黄色葡萄球菌和大肠杆菌 18~24h 的混合培养液。

(2) 普通琼脂平板培养基、接种环、酒精灯、温箱等。

【实验方法】

分区划线分离法

(1) 烧灼接种环以灭菌，冷却后，于混合培养液中取一环菌液。

(2) 左手持琼脂平板，打开皿盖一边数厘米，将菌液涂抹在平板表面左侧边缘部分。烧灼接种环，冷却，自涂抹部分开始，连续平行或蛇形划线，直至平板的 1/4，为 1 区（划线时接种环与培养基表面约呈 45°）。

(3) 再次烧灼接种环，待冷，转动皿底 45°，依次在平板 2、3、4、5 区划线接种。每划完一个区域是否需要对接种环进行烧灼灭菌视标本中含菌量而定。每一区的划线与上区交叉接触，每区线间保持一定距离，密而不重叠，如此形成后一区菌量少于前一区

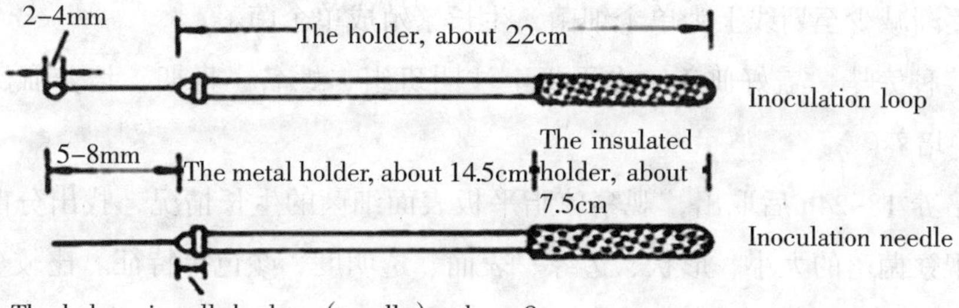


Figure 15 Inoculation Loop and Inoculation Needle

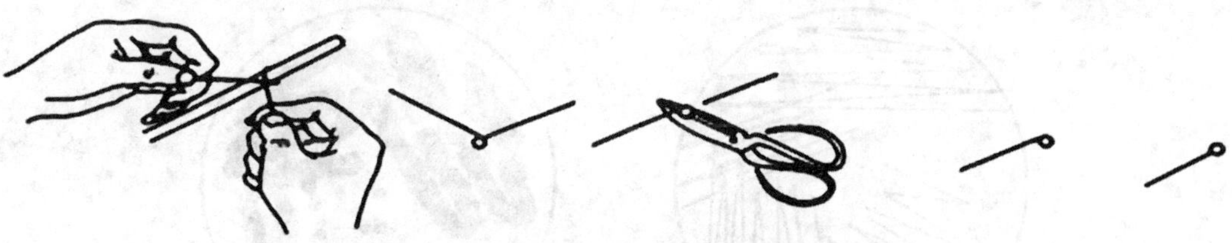

Figure 16 The Procedure of Making an Inoculation Loop

(2) Usage: Grasp the inoculation loop (needle) with thumb, index finger and middle finger of your right hand, just like holding a pen. Pass the metal wire through the outer flame of the alcohol lamp and heat it to redness to sterilize it. Then flame the metal holder twice quickly to kill the bacteria on the surface. Let it cool down before use. After using, flame the proximal portion which has a little distance from the wire, waiting for the heat conducted to the loop (needle) and the water on the surface evaporated. Then flame the inoculation loop (needle), and put it on the rack. Do not put it everywhere, avoiding burning the experiment table or other items.

(3) Application: Inoculation loops are used for streak inoculation, transferring pure cultures and smear preparation. Inoculation needles are used for stab inoculation and selecting individual colonies.

**【Materials and Equipment】**

(1) Bacteria: Mixed culture of *Staphylococcus aureus* and *Escherichia coli* which is cultured for 18–24h.

(2) General agar plate medium, inoculation loop, alcohol lamp, thermostat, etc.

**【Methods】**

Sectional streak method

(1) Flame the inoculation loop to ensure sterilization, allow the loop to cool down and take a loop of the mixed culture.

(2) Hold the agar plate with your left hand, lift the lid just enough to insert the loop, smear the mixed culture on the left edge of the agar plate. Flame the loop to ensure sterilization and cool it, streak this small sample in a zig-zag horizontal pattern until 1/4 of the plate is covered. It's the area 1 (take the loop and hold it at a 45° angle from the plate).

(3) Flame the loop to kill the remaining bacteria on the loop. Cool the loop. Rotate the

的情形，逐渐减少至划线上为单个细菌，生长繁殖成单个菌落。

(4) 接种完毕，盖好皿盖，在平板上注明班组、姓名、日期，培养皿倒放，置于37℃温箱中培养。

(5) 培养 18~24h 后取出，观察琼脂平板表面细菌的生长情况，找出分散的单个菌落。仔细观察菌落的大小、形状、边缘、表面、透明度、颜色等特征。比较金黄色葡萄球菌和大肠杆菌菌落特征的差异。（图 17）

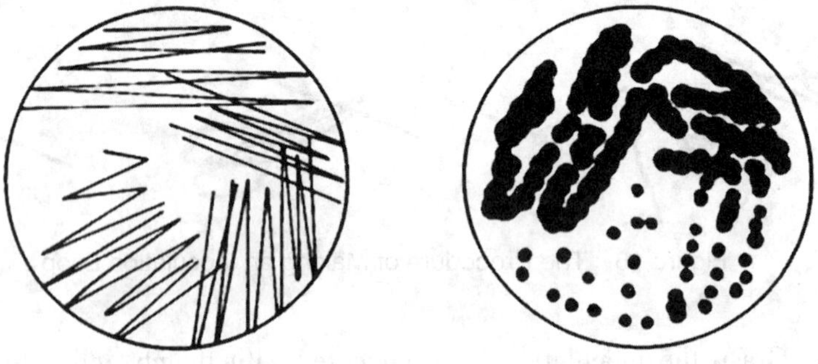

图 17 分区划线法（左）及菌落分布示意图（右）

**【实验结果】**

琼脂平板表面分布两种菌落：金黄色葡萄球菌菌落为金黄色圆形突起的小菌落，表面光滑湿润，边缘整齐，不透明；大肠杆菌菌落为灰白色圆形，略突起，中等大小，边缘整齐，光滑湿润，不透明。

## （二）细菌纯培养接种法

**【实验原理】**

分离到纯种细菌后，常需接种至各种有关培养基，以进一步测试其生化反应等生物学性状。根据培养基的物理状态不同，纯种接种法有斜面培养基接种法、液体培养基接种法和半固体穿刺接种法三种。斜面培养基接种法主要用于纯培养及保存菌种；液体培养基接种法用于增菌培养；半固体穿刺接种法用于保存菌种，观察细菌的动力和生化反应。

**【实验器材】**

(1) 菌种：大肠杆菌 18~24h 琼脂斜面培养物。

(2) 培养基：琼脂斜面培养基、液体培养基。

(3) 酒精灯、接种环、接种针、温箱。

plate about 45 degrees and spread the bacteria from the end of the last streak into area 2, 3, 4 and 5 using the same motion in step 2. Whether flame the loop or not depends on the number of the bacteria. As you move from one quadrant to another, there is a step-wise dilution of the original culture across the entire available surface. The quadrant with which you begin shows dense bacteria, whereas the last quadrant shows the presence of isolated single bacterium which will grow into individual colonies.

(4) After the inoculation is finished, place the lid back and invert the plate. Label the plate with your group, your name and the date. Then put the plate in 37℃ thermostat.

(5) Incubate the plate for 18–24 hours. Observe the bacterial growth situation and find the scattered individual colonies. Observe the characteristics of the bacterial colonies: size, shape, margin, surface, transparency and color, etc. Distinguish the difference of the colony characteristics between *Staphylococcus aureus* and *Escherichia coli*. (Figure 17)

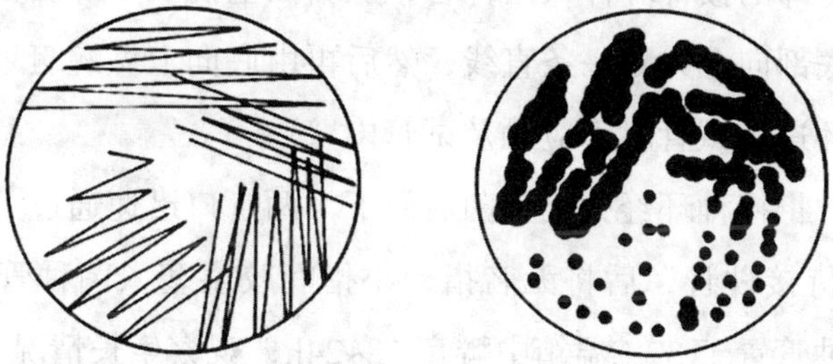

Figure 17 Sectional Streak Method (left) and the Bacterial Colony Model (right)

**【Results】**

There are two kinds of colonies on the argar plate. *Staphylococcus aureus* colonies demonstrate circular shape, golden yellow color, and are convex with smooth and moist surface and entire margins, not transparent. *Escherichia coli* colonies exhibit pale color in round shape, which have middle size, entire margin, smooth and moist and are slightly raised and not transparent.

## 2. Inoculation Methods for Pure Culture

**【Principle】**

Now that you have a pure bacterial culture, you need to transfer it to distinct culture mediums to test its biochemical and other biological characteristics. Inoculation methods can be classified into three ways based on physical properties of the medium: inoculation on slant medium, inoculation in liquid medium and stab inoculation on the semisolid medium. The first way is available in pure culture and storing bacteria. The second way is used for bacterial proliferation. And the last way is designed to store bacteria, observe the bacterial dynamics and biochemistry reaction.

**【Materials and Equipment】**

(1) Bacteria: *Escherichia coli* culture on agar slant medium incubated for 18–24 hours.

(2) Medium: agar slant medium, liquid medium.

**【实验方法】**

1. 斜面培养基接种法

(1) 左手拇指、食指、中指及无名指分别握持菌种管与待接种的培养基管，使菌种管位于外侧，培养基管位于内侧。斜面部分均应向上，管口稍高，以免管底凝固水浸湿培养基表面。

(2) 右手拇指、食指先转动两管胶塞，以便接种时易于拔取。

(3) 右手持接种环，烧灼灭菌，柄部也要迅速通过火焰2~3次以杀灭表面的杂菌，灭菌后拿在手中，勿与其他物品接触。

(4) 以右手无名指与小指拔取菌种管胶塞，再用手掌与小指拔取待接种管胶塞，随后将两管管口迅速通过火焰灭菌。

(5) 将灭菌后冷却的接种环伸入菌种管，从斜面上挑取少许菌苔，退出管后再伸入待接种管，自斜面底部向上先划一条直线，然后再由底向上做蜿蜒划线（勿触破培养基表面，粘菌的接种环进出试管时不应触及试管内壁）。

(6) 接种完毕，将接种环经火焰灭菌后放下。两管口迅速通过火焰2~3次灭菌，先将指掌间胶塞塞入待接种管，后将无名指、小指间胶塞塞入菌种管。将菌种管放回原处。标记后，将接种管置于37℃温箱中孵育18~24h，观察生长情况。

2. 液体培养基接种法

(1) 左手握持菌种管及肉汤管。

(2) 将接种环经火焰灭菌后，伸入菌种管取少量菌苔，再伸入肉汤管中，在接近上液面的管壁上轻轻研磨，使细菌混于肉汤中。

(3) 接种完毕，将接种环灭菌后放下。分别塞好胶塞（方法同前）置于37℃温箱中孵育18~24h，观察生长情况。

3. 半固体穿刺接种法

(1) 左手握持菌种管及待接种管（方法同前）。

(2) 右手持接种针，经火焰灭菌后，挑取少许菌苔，于待接种培养基中心垂直插入接近管底处，然后转动接种针，原路退出。

(3) 接种完毕，接种针灭菌后放下，分别塞好胶塞。做好标记后，将接种管置于37℃温箱中孵育18~24h，观察有无细菌生长，细菌有无动力。

(3) Alcohol lamp, inoculation loop, inoculation needle, thermostat.

【**Methods**】

### 1. Inoculation on slant medium

(1) Hold the bacterial tube and the tube to be inoculated with the thumb, index finger, middle finger and ring finger of your left hand, keep the tube to be inoculated be inner side of the bacterial tube. Make sure that the slant toward upside to avoid water soaking the surface of the medium.

(2) Rotate the plugs of both tubes with the thumb and index finger of your right hand to make it easier to remove.

(3) Take the inoculation loop with your right hand, and flame it for sterilization. Then flame the metal holder twice or three times quickly to kill the bacteria on the surface. After sterilization, hold it in your hand, and take far away from other items.

(4) Remove the plug of the bacterial tube with ring finger and little finger of your right hand, then remove the plug of the tube to be inculated with your plam and little finger. Flame the mouths of the two tubes for sterilization.

(5) Insert the sterile inoculation loop into the bacterial tube to obtain a small amount of bacteria. Withdraw the inoculation loop and place it on the agar slant's surface at the bottom of the tube to be inculated. Move the inoculation loop in a zig-zag pattern as you pull it upward out of the tube (Do not damage the medium. Do not touch the inner wall of the tubes with the inoculation loop)

(6) After finish inoculating, flame the inoculation loop and lay it down. Flame the mouths of both tubes for 2–3 times. Place the plug of the tube to be inoculated back and then place the plug of the bacterial tube back. Put the bacterial tube back. Label the tube to be inoculated and incubate it for 18–24 hours in a thermostat at 37℃. Examine the tube for the bacterial growth.

### 2. Inoculation in liquid medium

(1) Hold the bacterial tube and the broth tube with your left hand.

(2) Flame the inoculation loop, then take a small amount of bacterial colony from the bacterial tube with it. Mix the loop of bacterial culture into the broth tube by grinding the baeterial colony lightly on the inner wall of the broth tube.

(3) After finish inoculating, flame the inoculation inoculation loop and lay it down. Place the plugs of the tubes back in the same way above. Label the tube to be inoculated and incubate it for 18–24 hours in a thermostat at 37℃. Examine the tube for the bacterial growth.

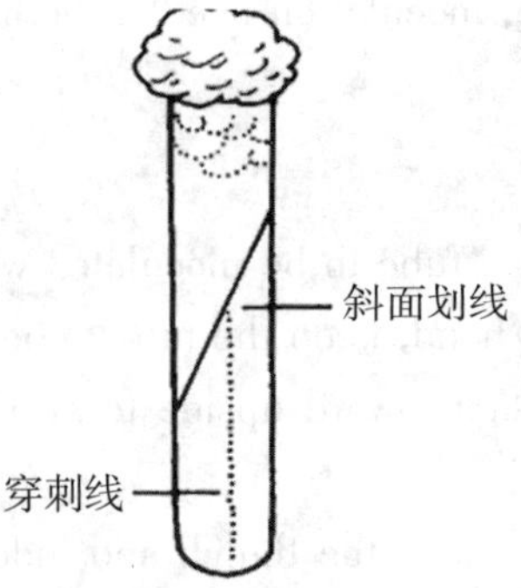

图 18 斜面培养基接种法

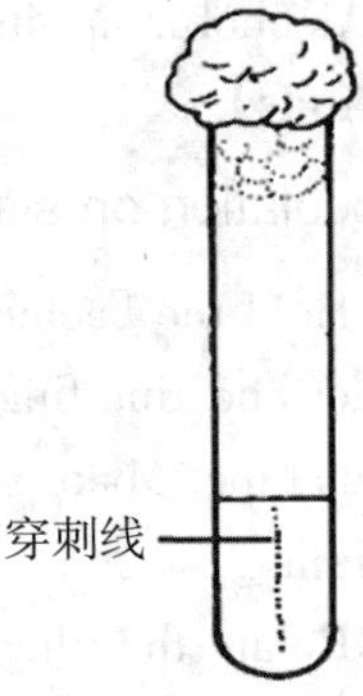

图 19 半固体穿刺接种法

**【实验结果】**

细菌种类不同，在培养基上的生长状态也不相同。通过观察细菌的生长状态，有助于鉴定细菌。

(1) 斜面上生长状态观察：可见有均匀一致的菌苔，如有不同的菌落出现，则表明受污染了，有杂菌存在。

(2) 液体培养基中生长状态观察：培养前的液体培养基多为清澈透明的。接种细菌后由于细菌种类不同，可有以下三种生长形式：

①混浊：液体变为混浊。

②菌膜：液体澄清，液体表面有一薄膜。

③沉淀：液体较澄清，管底有沉淀物。

(3) 半固体中生长状态观察：无鞭毛（无运动）的细菌，经培养后仅沿穿刺线生长，培养基清亮。有鞭毛（能运动）的细菌，沿穿刺线向外扩散，穿刺线模糊不清，培养基混浊。

**【思考题】**

(1) 细菌生长繁殖需要的基本条件有哪些?

(2) 细菌分离培养的方法有哪些?

## 二、细菌生化反应

不同种或型别的细菌，因为其形态和菌落特点基本相同，所以只依靠对形态和菌落的观察，不能加以区别。但是由于不同种型的细菌所具有的酶系统各不相同，对营养物质的利用能力各异，因而在代谢过程中所产生的代谢产物也不同。应用生物化学方法检测细菌的代谢产物，有助于细菌属、种的鉴定。这种利用生化方法来鉴别细菌的实验，统称为细菌生化反应，是鉴定细菌的重要方法之一。

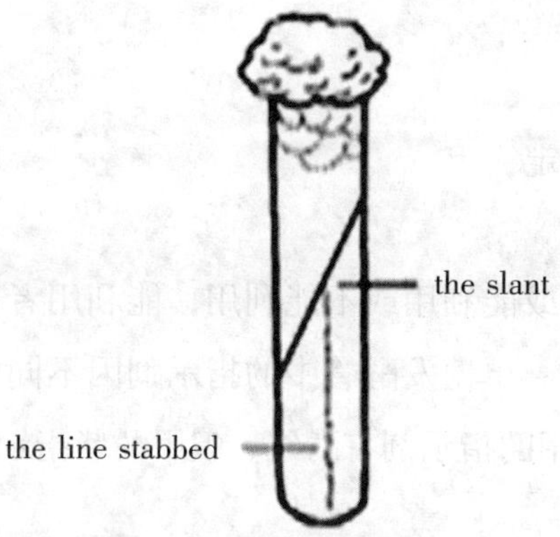


Figure 18 Inoculation on Slant Medium

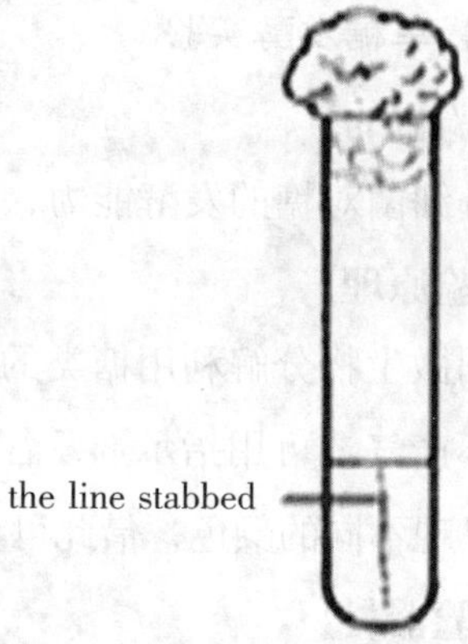


Figure 19 Stab Inoculation on the Semisolid Medium

### 3. Stab inoculation on the semisolid medium

(1) Hold the bacterial tube and the tube to be inoculated with your left hand.

(2) Hold the inoculation needle with your right hand and flame it. Pick a small amount of bacteria, insert the inoculation needle without touching the sides of the tube and continue downward until the needle nearly reaches the bottom of the tube. Rotate the needle and then withdraw from the tube by the same route slowly.

(3) After finish inoculating, flame the inoculation needle and lay it down. Replace the plugs of the tubes in the same way above. Label the tube to be inoculated and incubate it for 18 –24 hours in a thermostat at 37℃. Examine the tube for the bacterial growth and its motility.

**【Results】**

Different bacteria will exhibit varying growth characteristics on the culture medium. These growth patterns can be used to aid in identifying an unknown bacterium.

(1) The growth on the slant: Each colony should have the same appearance. If you find different bacterial colonies, it may be a sign of contamination.

(2) The growth in the liquid medium: The liquid medium is always transparent before incubation. There are three different growth patterns after incubation:

①Turbid: The liquid turns turbid.

②Pellicle: The liquid is transparent and there is a pellicle on the surface.

③Sediment: The liquid appears a little transparent, but there is some sediment at the bottom of the tube.

(3) The growth on the semisolid medium: The bacteria without flagella grow along the line stabbed, and the medium is clear. The bacteria with flagella can move and spread along the line stabbed, the line stabbed is fuzzy and the medium is turbid.

**【Questions】**

(1) What are the basic conditions for the growth and proliferation of bacteria?

(2) What are the methods of bacterial isolation and culture?

### （一）单糖发酵实验

**【实验目的】**

检查细菌对糖的发酵能力，从而对细菌进行鉴定。

**【实验原理】**

不同微生物分解利用糖类的能力有很大差异，或能利用或不能利用，能利用者，或产气或不产气。可用指示剂及各种发酵管进行检测。单糖发酵管中的指示剂因不同的酸碱度而呈现不同的颜色，借此可鉴别细菌。一般常用的指示剂有酚红、嗅甲酚紫指示剂。

**【实验器材】**

(1) 菌种：大肠杆菌、伤寒杆菌琼脂斜面 18~24h 培养物。

(2) 葡萄糖、乳糖发酵管（含 1%糖，以溴甲酚紫为指示剂）。

(3) 酒精灯、接种环、接种针、温箱。

**【实验方法】**

(1) 大肠杆菌、伤寒杆菌各接种 1 支葡萄糖和 1 支乳糖发酵管。

(2) 置于 37℃温箱中培养 18~24h 后，观察结果。

**【实验结果】**

单糖发酵管颜色未改变时，说明细菌不分解该糖，用“–”表示；当紫色变成黄色时，说明细菌分解该糖，用“+”表示；当培养基不仅变黄而且倒置小管中有气泡产生时，说明细菌分解该糖既产酸又产气，用“⊕”表示。

### （二）V–P 实验（Voges-Proskauer Test）

**【实验原理】**

某些细菌可分解葡萄糖产生丙酮酸，丙酮酸脱羧生成乙酰甲基甲醇，在碱性环境中被氧化为二乙酰，再与培养基中精氨酸的胍基结合，生成红色化合物，培养基变红色，则实验结果为阳性，记为“+”；培养基不变色，则实验结果为阴性，记为“–”。

**【实验器材】**

(1) 大肠杆菌、产气杆菌 18~24h 培养物。

(2) 葡萄糖蛋白胨水培养基。

(3) V–P 试剂：甲液（6%萘酚酒精溶液）、乙液（40%KOH 溶液）。

(4) 酒精灯、接种环、接种针、温箱。

**【实验方法】**

分别将大肠杆菌、产气杆菌斜面培养物接种于葡萄糖蛋白胨水培养基中，置于 37℃温箱中培养 48h，取出后于每 2mL 培养液中分别加入 V–P 试剂甲液 1mL，混匀，再加 V–P 试剂乙液 4mL，充分振摇，静置 5~15min，观察结果。

## ii . Biochemical Reaction of Bacteria

Different species or types of bacteria cannot be distinguished by observation of their morphology or colony characteristics alone, because they are basically the same. However, because the different types of bacteria have different enzyme systems and different ability of using nutrients, so their metabolites are always different. Detection of bacterial metabolites by biochemical methods would be helpful to identify the genus and species of bacteria. The experiment using biochemical method to identify bacteria, collectively referred as the biochemical reaction, is one of the most important methods for the identification of bacteria.

### 1. Monosaccharide Fermentation Test

**【Aim】**

Examine the ability of bacteria to ferment sugar, thus to identify bacteria.

**【Principle】**

Different types of microbes have significant differences in the ability of decomposing sugars, such as being able to use sugar or not, and the former producing gas or not. Indicators and various fermentation tubes can be used to test them. We can identify bacteria by different colors the indicator shows in the monosaccharide fermentation tubes because of different pH value. The commonly used indicators are phenol red and bromocresol purple.

**【Materials and Equipment】**

(1) Bacteria: cultures of *Escherichia coli* and *Bacillus typhi* which are cultured on the agar slant medium for 18–24h.

(2) Glucose, lactose fermentation tubes (containing 1% sugar, indicator is bromocresol purple).

(3) Alcohol lamp, inoculation loop, inoculation needle, thermostat.

**【Methods】**

(1) Inoculate *Escherichia coli* and *Bacillus typhi* in one glucose and lactose fermentation tube, respectively.

(2) Incubate at 37℃ in the thermostat for 18–24h, then observe the result.

**【Results】**

If the color in the monosaccharide fermentation tube does not change, it indicates that the bacteria do not decompose sugar. Represent it with a "–". If the purple turns to yellow, it indicates that the bacteria decompose sugar. Represent it with a "+". If the medium not only becomes yellow, but also gets bubbles in a small inverted tube, it indicates that the bacteria can decompose sugar and produce gas. Represent it with a "⊕".

### 2. Voges-Proskauer Test

**【Principle】**

Some bacteria can decompose glucose into pyruvic acid, then pyruvic acid decarboxylates into acetyl methyl carbinol. In the alkaline environment, they are oxidized to be diacetyl, which can combine with the guanidyl of arginine in the culture medium to produce red

【实验结果】

产气杆菌管出现红色，为 V–P 实验阳性；大肠杆菌管无色，为 V–P 实验阴性。

（三）甲基红实验

【实验原理】

某些细菌可以分解葡萄糖产生丙酮酸，丙酮酸进而分解为甲酸、乙酸、乳酸等，使培养基 pH 值降低至 4.5，加入甲基红指示剂呈红色，为甲基红实验阳性。若产酸量少或所产生的酸进一步转化为醇、醛、酮、气体和水，则培养基 pH 值高于 5.4，加入甲基红指示剂呈黄色，为阴性。

【实验器材】

（1）大肠杆菌、产气杆菌 18~24h 培养物。

（2）葡萄糖蛋白胨水培养基。

（3）甲基红指示剂。

（4）酒精灯、接种环、接种针、温箱。

【实验方法】

分别将大肠杆菌、产气杆菌斜面培养物接种于葡萄糖蛋白胨水培养基中，置于 37℃温箱中培养 48h，取出后分别滴加甲基红指示剂 2 滴，混匀后观察结果。

【实验结果】

大肠杆菌管呈红色，为甲基红实验阳性；产气杆菌管出现黄色，为甲基红实验阴性。

（四）枸橼酸盐利用实验

【实验原理】

某些细菌能利用枸橼酸盐作为碳源，并分解枸橼酸盐生成碳酸盐，使培养基变为碱性，培养基中的指示剂——麝香草酚蓝由绿色转为深蓝色，为枸橼酸盐利用实验阳性。

【实验器材】

（1）大肠杆菌、产气杆菌 18~24h 培养物。

（2）枸橼酸盐培养基：含枸橼酸钠、磷酸二氢铵、磷酸氢二钾、氯化钠、麝香草酚蓝等。

（3）酒精灯、接种环、接种针、温箱。

【实验方法】

分别将大肠杆菌、产气杆菌培养物接种于枸橼酸盐培养基中，置于 37℃温箱中培养 24h 后，取出观察结果。

【实验结果】

产气杆菌管培养基斜面出现菌苔，呈现蓝色，为枸橼酸盐利用实验阳性；大肠杆菌

compounds. If the culture medium turns red, it indicates that the test is positive and represent it with a "+". On the contrary, it indicates negative, and represent it with a "−".

**【Materials and Equipment】**

(1) Cultures of *Escherichia coli, Enterobacter aerogenes* which are cultured for 18–24h. (2) Glucose peptone water medium.

(3) V–P reagents: A solution (6% naphthol alcohol solution), B solution (40% KOH solution).

(4) Alcohol lamp, inoculation loop, inoculation needle, thermostat.

**【Methods】**

Inoculate slant cultures of *Escherichia coli* and *Enterobacter aerogenes* into glucose peptone water medium, respectively. Incubate in 37℃ thermostat for 48h. Take 2mL of culture and mix with 1mL A solution of V–P reagent. Mix and then add 4mL B solution of V–P reagent. Shake fully and observe the result after stand for 5–15min.

**【Results】**

The color in the *Enterobacter aerogenes* tube turns red, it's positive result in V–P test, while the *Escherichia coli* is negative result for the tube remains colorless.

### 3. Methyl Red Test

**【Principle】**

Some bacteria can decompose glucose into pyruvic acid, and then pyruvic acid decomposes into formic acid, acetic acid, lactic acid, etc, which make the pH value of medium reduces to 4.5. Add methyl red indicator, the color of medium turns red, it indicates that the test is positive. If the generated acid is less or further converts to alcohol, aldehyde, ketone, gas and water, the medium's pH is higher than 5.4, when add methyl red indicator, it will turn yellow, meaning the test is negative.

**【Materials and Equipment】**

(1) Cultures of *Escherichia coli, Enterobacter aerogenes* which are cultured for 18–24h. (2) Glucose peptone water medium.

(3) Methyl red indicator.

(4) Alcohol lamp, inoculation loop, inoculation needle, thermostat.

**【Methods】**

Inoculate slant cultures of *Escherichia coli* and *Enterobacter aerogenes* into glucose peptone water medium, respectively. Culture them in 37℃ thermostat for 48h. Then add two drops of methyl red indicator, respectively. Mix and observe the result.

**【Results】**

The *Escherichia coli* tube turns red which indicates the methyl red test is positive. The *Enterobacter aerogenes* tube appears yellow, so the test is negative.

### 4. Citrate Utilization Test

**【Principle】**

Some bacteria can use citrate as carbon source, and decompose it into carbonate. Thus

管未见菌苔，呈绿色，为枸橼酸盐利用实验阴性。

（五）靛基质（吲哚）实验

【实验原理】

有些细菌具有色氨酸酶，能分解蛋白胨中的色氨酸而产生无色靛基质（吲哚），与滴加的靛基质试剂（对二甲基氨基苯甲醛）于培养基的液面上形成红色复合物——吲哚者，为吲哚阳性反应，仍呈黄色者为阴性反应。

【实验器材】

(1) 大肠杆菌、产气杆菌 18~24h 培养物。

(2) 蛋白胨水培养基、靛基质试剂（对二甲基氨基苯甲醛）。

(3) 酒精灯、接种环、接种针、温箱。

【实验方法】

分别将大肠杆菌、产气杆菌培养物接种于蛋白胨水培养基中，置于 37℃温箱中培养 18~24h，每管沿管壁加靛基质试剂 2~3 滴，使试剂浮于培养物表面（不能摇匀），即刻观察结果。

【实验结果】

大肠杆菌管中两液面交界处形成玫瑰红色吲哚，为阳性反应；产气杆菌管中无变化，为阴性反应。

（六）硫化氢实验

【实验原理】

某些细菌能分解培养基中的含硫氨基酸（如胱氨酸），生成硫化氢，与培养基中的铁盐或铅盐形成硫化亚铁或硫化铅，呈黑色，为阳性反应。培养基颜色无变化，则为阴性反应。

【实验器材】

(1) 大肠杆菌、变形杆菌 18~24h 培养物。

(2) 醋酸铅培养基。

(3) 酒精灯、接种环、接种针、温箱。

【实验方法】

分别将大肠杆菌、变形杆菌培养物接种于醋酸铅培养基中，置于 37℃温箱中培养 18~24h 后，观察结果。

【实验结果】

变形杆菌培养管穿刺部位呈黑褐色，为阳性反应；大肠杆菌培养管颜色无变化，为阴性反应。

the medium becomes alkaline. If the indicator—thymol blue makes the medium turn from green to dark blue, it indicates that the test is positive.

**【Materials and Equipment】**

(1) Cultures of *Escherichia coli*, *Enterobacter aerogenes* which are cultured for 18 to 24h.

(2) Citrate medium: contains sodium citrate, ammonium dihydrogen phosphate, dipotassium phosphate, sodium chloride, thymol blue, etc.

(3) Alcohol lamp, inoculation loop, inoculation needle, thermostat.

**【Methods】**

Inoculate cultures of *Escherichia coli* and *Enterobacter aerogenes* on citrate medium, respectively. Incubate them in 37℃ thermostat for 24h. Then observe it.

**【Results】**

In the *Enterobacter aerogenes* tube, there grows bacterial lawn on the slant medium and the color turns blue, it indicates that the test is positive. And there is no bacterial lawn and the medium remains green in the *Escherichia coli* tube, meaning the test is negative.

### 5. Indole Test

**【Principle】**

Some bacteria have tryptophanase which can decompose tryptophan in peptone into colorless indole. Then a red complex—indole can be formed at the medium surface when add some indole reagent because of the reaction between indole and indole reagent (P-dimethylamino benzaldehyde). This indicates that the test is positive. If the color is still yellow, the test is negative.

**【Materials and Equipment】**

(1) Cultures of *Escherichia coli*, *Enterobacter aerogenes* which are cultured for 18–24h.

(2) Peptone water medium, indole reagent (P-dimethylamino benzaldehyde).

(3) Alcohol lamp, inoculation loop, inoculation needle, thermostat.

**【Methods】**

Inoculate cultures of *Escherichia coli* and *Enterobacter aerogenes* into peptone water medium, respectively. Incubate them in 37℃ thermostat for 18–24h. Then add two to three drops of indole reagent along the wall of the tube, making the reagent float on the surface of the culture (do not shake). Observe the result immediately.

**【Results】**

There is rose red indole formed at liquid junction in the *Escherichia coli* tube, which indicates that the result of indole test is positive. But the *Enterobacter aerogenes* tube has no change, and the test is negative.

### 6. Hydrogen Sulfide Test

**【Principle】**

Some bacteria can decompose the sulfur-containing amino acids in the medium (such as cystine) into hydrogen sulfide, which reacts with iron or lead salt in the medium and generates black iron monosulfide or lead monosulfide, and causes the medium turning black,

### （七）尿素分解实验

**【实验原理】**

某些细菌具有尿素分解酶，能分解尿素，产生大量的氨，使培养基变碱性，酚红指示剂呈紫红色，为阳性反应；不变色者为阴性反应。

**【实验器材】**

（1）痢疾杆菌、变形杆菌 18~24h 培养物。

（2）尿素培养基：含尿素、蛋白胨、氯化钠、酚红指示剂等。

（3）酒精灯、接种环、接种针、温箱。

**【实验方法】**

分别将痢疾杆菌、变形杆菌培养物接种于尿素培养基中，置于 37℃温箱中培养 18~24h 后，观察结果。

**【实验结果】**

变形杆菌培养基呈紫红色，为阳性反应；痢疾杆菌培养基不变色，为阴性反应。

**【思考题】**

什么叫细菌的生化反应？有何应用？

which indicats the hydrogen sulfide test is positive. If the color of the medium does not change, the test is negative.

**【Materials and Equipment】**

(1) Cultures of *Escherichia coli*, *Bacillus proteus* which are cultured for 18 to 24h.

(2) Lead acetate medium.

(3) Alcohol lamp, inoculation loop, inoculation needle, thermostat.

**【Methods】**

Inoculate the cultures of *Escherichia coli* and *Bacillus proteus* into lead acetate medium, respectively. Incubate them in 37℃ thermostat for 18–24h and observe the result.

**【Results】**

The stabbed part of *Bacillus proteus* culture tube is black brown, indicating the test is positive. The *Escherichia coli* tube has no change, meaning the test is negative.

### 7. Urea Hydrolysis Test

**【Principle】**

Some bacteria have the urease which can hydrolyze urea into large amounts of ammonia, so the medium becomes alkaline. If the indicator—phenol red turns purple red, it indicates that the test is positive, or the test is negative.

**【Materials and Equipment】**

(1) Cultures of *Bacillus dysenteriae*, *Bacillus proteus* which are cultured for 18 to 24h.

(2) Urea medium: contains urea, peptone, sodium chloride, phenol red indicator, etc.

(3) Alcohol lamp, inoculation loop, inoculation needle, thermostat.

**【Methods】**

Inoculate cultures of *Bacillus dysenteriae* and *Bacillus proteus* on urea medium, respectively. Incubate them in 37℃ incubator for 18–24h. Then observe the result.

**【Results】**

The *Bacillus proteus* tube appears purple red, which indicates that the test is positive. The color of *Bacillus dysenteriae* tube has no change, the test is negative.

**【Questions】**

What are the biochemical reactions of bacteria? What is the application?

# 实验十四 细菌的分布

## 一、自然环境中细菌的检查

**【实验原理】**

自然界中分布着大量微生物，包括各种细菌、真菌等。通过本实验了解细菌分布的广泛性及细菌培养技术。

### （一）空气中细菌的检查

**【实验目的】**

了解微生物在空气中的分布。

**【实验器材】**

⑴ 普通琼脂平板培养基。

⑵ 酒精灯、接种环、温箱。

**【实验方法】**

⑴ 取普通琼脂平板培养基 4 个，其中 3 个去盖，置于不同的环境中（实验桌上、走廊、窗台），在空气中暴露 15~30min，盖好皿盖。另外 1 个不去盖，作为阴性对照。

⑵ 标记班组、姓名，置于 37℃温箱中培养 18~24h 后，取出观察结果。

**【实验结果】**

对照平板培养基上无菌落生长，去盖的 3 个平板培养基表面有不同数目的菌落生长，比较菌落数的差异及其特征，并分析原因。

### （二）水中细菌的检查

**【实验目的】**

了解微生物在水中的分布。

**【实验器材】**

⑴ 高层琼脂培养基、水标本、无菌生理盐水。

⑵ 无菌试管、吸管、空培养皿、细菌菌落计数器。

# XIV. The Distribution of Bacteria

## ⅰ. Bacterial Examination in the Natural Environment

**【Principle】**

A large number of microorganisms distribute in nature, including bacteria, fungi, and so on. Understand the wide distribution of bacteria and bacterial culture techniques through this experiment.

### 1. The Examination of Bacteria in the Air

**【Aim】**

Get to know the distribution of bacteria in the air.

**【Materials and Equipment】**

(1) Ordinary agar plate mediums.

(2) Alcohol lamp, inoculation loop, thermostat.

**【Methods】**

(1) Take four ordinary agar plate mediums, open the covers of three plate mediums and place them at three different sites (on the bench, on the corridor and on the window sill), respectively. After exposing to air at different places for 15–30min, cover the mediums. Do not open the cover of the 4th medium and use it as a negative control.

(2) Label class, team and individual name, put the four agar plate mediums in the thermostat at 37℃, incubate for 18–24h, then observe the result.

**【Results】**

No colonies grow in the control plate medium, on the surface of other three plate mediums, a different number of colonies grow. Compare the differences of numbers and features of colonies, and analyze the reasons.

### 2. The Examination of Bacteria in the Water

**【Aim】**

To understand the distribution of bacteria in the water.

**【Materials and Equipment】**

(1) Top agar medium, water specimen, normal saline.

(2) Sterile tubes, pipettes, culture dishes, the bacterial colony counter.

(3) 酒精灯、接种环、温箱。

【实验方法】

吸取 1mL 水标本加入无菌空培养皿中，将高层琼脂培养基加热溶化，冷却到 60℃左右，注入培养皿中，立即混匀，冷凝后，置于 37℃温箱中培养 18~24h 后，取出观察结果。

【实验结果】

对菌落进行计数，即每毫升水样品中的细菌总数。

## 二、正常人体的细菌检查

### (一) 皮肤细菌的检查

【实验目的】

了解微生物在人体皮肤表面的分布。

【实验原理】

在人体的体表和人体与外界相通的腔道中，都有一定量的细菌存在，在正常情况下不致病，这些细菌通过直接取标本染色或经过培养可以检出。

【实验器材】

(1) 普通琼脂平板培养基、2%碘酒、75%酒精。

(2) 酒精灯、接种环、接种针、温箱。

【实验方法】

取普通琼脂平板培养基一个，用蜡笔在背面分成三格，标记为 1、2、3，先将手指在 1 处按指纹，然后将手指用碘酒或 75%酒精消毒后在 2 处按指纹，留 3 处作为空白对照。标记班组、姓名后，置于 37℃温箱中培养 18~24h 后，取出观察结果。

【实验结果】

琼脂平板培养基 1 处见大小不等、形态各异的菌落生长，2 处无或有很少菌落生长，3 处无细菌生长。

### (二) 咽部细菌的检查

【实验目的】

了解微生物在人体咽部的分布。

【实验器材】

血琼脂平板培养基、无菌棉拭子、接种环、酒精灯、温箱。

【实验方法】

用无菌棉拭子在咽部取分泌物，涂在血琼脂平板一端，用接种环作分离划线接种，

(3) Alcohol lamp, inoculation loop, thermostat.

**【Methods】**

Add 1mL water specimen to a sterile dish, melt the top agar medium and cool it to about 60℃, pour it into the dish, immediately mix. After condensed, incubate it in the thermostat for 18–24h at 37℃ and then observe the result.

**【Results】**

Count the number of colonies, and it is the total number of bacteria in the water specimen per 1mL.

## ii. Normal Human Bacterial Examination

### 1. Detection of Bacteria on Human Skin

**【Aim】**

To know the distribution of microorganisms on the surface of human skin.

**【Principle】**

On the surface of human body, and in the cavities linked with the outside world, there is a certain amount of bacteria. Under normal circumstances, these bacteria do not cause diseases, and can be detected through direct staining or culture.

**【Materials and Equipment】**

(1) Ordinary agar plate medium, 2% iodine, 75% alcohol.

(2) Alcohol lamp, inoculation loop, inoculation needle, thermostat.

**【Methods】**

Take an ordinary agar plate, divide it into three areas on the back with crayon, label as 1, 2, and 3. On the surface of area 1, print a fingerprint with a finger. After disinfect this finger with iodine or 75% alcohol, print a fingerprint on area 2. Area 3 acts as a blank control and do not touch it. After label class, team and individual name, incubate it in the thermostat at 37℃ for 18–24h and then observe the result.

**【Results】**

On area 1, there are many colonies growing with different sizes and shapes. There is no or few colonies growing on area 2, and no colonies appear on area 3.

### 2. Detection of Bacteria in Pharyngeal Portion

**【Aim】**

To know the distribution of microorganisms at human pharyngeal portion.

**【Materials and Equipment】**

Blood agar plate medium, sterile cotton swab, inoculation loop, alcohol lamp, thermostat.

**【Methods】**

Take a little secretion in the throat with a sterile cotton swab, paint it on the edge of the blood agar plate medium and streak with an inoculation loop. Cover with lid and incubate in 37℃ thermostat for 18–24h, observe the result.

加盖后置于 37℃温箱中培养 18~24h 后，取出观察细菌生长情况。

**【实验结果】**

观察细菌的数量、种类等，注意是否有溶血环，并分析其意义。

**【Results】**

Observe the number and species of bacteria, etc. Note whether hemolytic rings appear, then analyze their significance.

# 实验十五　外界因素对细菌的影响

## 一、物理因素对细菌的影响

紫外线杀菌实验

【实验目的】

(1) 掌握紫外线杀菌的原理和方法。

(2) 熟悉紫外线杀菌的适用范围及应用中应注意的问题。

【实验原理】

紫外线的杀菌作用与波长有关，波长为240~280nm的紫外线有杀菌能力，其中，波长为265~266nm的紫外线杀菌作用最强。细菌DNA吸收了紫外线引起胸腺嘧啶形成二聚体，从而干扰了DNA的复制，轻则发生突变，重则导致死亡。紫外线杀菌力强而稳定，但穿透力弱，不能透过普通玻璃和有色纸张，因此，只适用于直接照射的物体表面消毒或空气消毒。

【实验器材】

(1) 大肠杆菌18~24h肉汤培养液。

(2) 普通琼脂平板培养基。

(3) 紫外线灯、酒精灯、接种环、温箱。

【实验方法】

(1) 取普通琼脂平板培养基一个，用蜡笔划分为二等份。用接种环取适量大肠杆菌密集划线接种，涂满1/2平板表面，空白的1/2作为对照。

(2) 将平板培养基放置在距紫外线60~100cm处，打开盖子，盖住平板的一半，直接受紫外线照射30min后，盖好盖子，置于37℃温箱，孵育18~24h后观察细菌生长情况。

【实验结果】

紫外线灯管直接照射处无细菌生长或仅有少量细菌生长，遮盖处有大量细菌生长。

# XV. The Influence of External Factors on Bacteria

## i. The Influence of Physical Factors on Bacteria

Ultraviolet Sterilization Experiment

**【Aim】**

(1) To master the principle and methods of ultraviolet sterilization.

(2) Get familiar with the applicable scope and problems of ultraviolet sterilization.

**【Principle】**

The function of ultraviolet sterilization has relation to its wavelength, of which those wavelength within 240–280nm have bactericidal ability and those wave length within 265–266nm have the strongest effect. Bacterial DNA absorbs UV and forms thymine dimer, which interferes with the DNA replication and causes different effects from mutation to death. Ultraviolet light shows strong and stable bactericidal effect. But its penetrating power is weak and cannot penetrate common glass and colored paper, so that it is only applicable for disinfection of objects' surfaces and air through direct illumination.

**【Materials and Equipment】**

(1) Broth culture of *Escherichia coli* which is cultured for 18–24h.

(2) Ordinary agar plate medium.

(3) Ultraviolet lamp, alcohol lamp, inoculation loop and thermostat.

**【Methods】**

(1) Take an ordinary agar plate medium and mark each part with a crayon after dividing it into two halves. Then inoculate a suitable amount of *Escherichia coli* on one half of the plate through dense streak by using inoculation loop, and the other part is blank control.

(2) Put the agar plate medium at 60–100cm away from ultraviolet ray and open the cover to shade half of the plate. After 30min of radiating, cover the plate and incubate in 37℃ thermostat for 18–24h, observe the growth of bacteria.

**【Results】**

There is no or little growth of bacteria in place directly illuminated by UV, while a large number of bacteria grow in the covered part.

## ii. The Influence of Chemical Factors on Bacteria

**【Principle】**

There are many kinds of chemical disinfectants with different bactericidal mechanisms,

## 二、化学因素对细菌的影响

【实验原理】

化学消毒剂的种类很多，杀菌机制因种类不同而异。主要通过使菌体蛋白变性或凝固，改变细胞膜的通透性，干扰细菌的代谢等方式，使细菌死亡。

【实验器材】

(1) 葡萄球菌、大肠杆菌 24h 肉汤培养液。

(2) 无菌琼脂平板培养基、无菌滤纸片、小镊子等。

(3) 2%碘酒、3%来苏水、1%龙胆紫、1:1 000 新洁尔灭。

(4) 酒精灯、接种环、温箱。

【实验方法】

(1) 取 2 个无菌琼脂平板培养基，用接种环分别取葡萄球菌及大肠杆菌数环，做来回划线接种，涂满琼脂平板培养基表面。

(2) 用无菌镊子取滤纸片各 2 张，分别浸于 2%碘酒、3%来苏水、1%龙胆紫、1:1 000 新洁尔灭四种消毒剂中，再将其分别等距离贴在两平板内相应的区域，置于 37℃温箱中孵育 24h 后，观察并测量纸片周围抑菌环直径的大小。

【实验结果】

消毒剂纸片周围抑菌环直径的大小表示该化学消毒剂杀菌作用的强弱。

## 三、细菌对抗生素的敏感性测定（琼脂扩散法）

抗菌药物是指具有杀菌和抑菌活性、用于预防和治疗微生物性感染的药物，包括抗生素和化学合成药物。前者是指对特异微生物有杀灭和抑制作用的微生物代谢产物，后者是经化学改造的半合成抗生素和化学合成药物。不同抗菌药物对病原微生物的杀菌或抑菌能力不同，不同病原微生物对同一抗菌药物的敏感性也不尽相同。通过抗菌药物敏感性实验（antimicrobial susceptibility test, AST）测定病原微生物对抗菌药物的敏感性，对临床治疗中选择合适的抗菌药物，及时控制感染有重要意义。

目前，进行抗菌药物敏感性实验（简称药敏实验）的方法主要有纸片扩散法、稀释法（包括肉汤稀释法和琼脂稀释法）、E 实验和自动化仪器等。下面介绍纸片扩散法和 E 实验。

### （一）纸片扩散法

【实验目的】

掌握纸片扩散法的原理、操作方法和结果的判读。

such as causing bacterial protein degeneration or solidification, changing the permeability of cell membrane, and interfering with the bacterial metabolism, etc.

**【Materials and Equipment】**

(1) Broth cultures of *Staphylococcus, Escherichia coli* which are cultured for 24h.

(2) The sterile agar plate medium, sterile filter paper, tweezers, etc.

(3) 2% iodine, 3% Lysol, 1% crystal violet, 1:1,000 bromogeramine.

(4) Alcohol lamp, inoculation loop and thermostat.

**【Methods】**

(1) Inoculate several rings of *Staphylococcus* and *Escherichia coli* on the whole surface of two sterile agar plate mediums, respectively through streak plate method.

(2) Immerse 2 pieces of filter paper in 2% iodine, 3% Lysol, 1% crystal violet, and 1:1,000 bromogeramine, respectively. Then take one of filter papers in each sanitizer with sterile forceps and paste them on *Staphylococcus* plate at corresponding sites. The other pieces of filter papers are pasted on *Escherichia coli* plate. Incubate the two plates in 37℃ thermostat for 24h and then observe the result, measure the diameter of the inhibition rings surrounding the papers.

**【Results】**

The diameter of the inhibition ring surrounding the filter paper represents the bactericidal effect of the chemical disinfectant.

## iii. Test on Bacterial Sensitivity to Antibiotics (Agar Diffusion Method)

Antimicrobial drugs have bactericidal and bacteriostatic activities which can be used for prevention and treatment of microbial infections, including antibiotics and chemical synthetic drugs. The former refers to some microbial metabolites which have functions of killing and inhibiting other special microbes. The latter refers to semi-synthetic antibiotics through chemical modification and chemical synthetic drugs. Different antimicrobial drugs have different abilities in killing or inhibiting a certain pathogenic microorganism, while different pathogenic microorganisms show different sensitivity to a certain antibacterial drug. Testing the sensitivity of pathogenic microorganisms to antimicrobial drugs through antimicrobial susceptibility test (AST) has important significance in choosing appropriate antimicrobial drugs in the clinical treatment and infection control.

At present, the methods of antimicrobial susceptibility test(abbreviation as drug sensitive test) include paper disk diffusion method, dilution method(includes the broth dilution method and agar dilution method), E test and automated instrument, etc. The following will introduce paper disk diffusion method and E test.

### 1. Paper Disk Diffusion Method

**【Aim】**

To master the principle, operation and result interpretation of paper disk diffusion method.

**【Principle】**

Paper disk diffusion method is a qualitative drug sensitivity determination method

【实验原理】

纸片扩散法是临床常用的药物敏感性定性测定方法，将含有定量抗菌药物的滤纸片贴在已接种测试菌的琼脂平板表面，纸片中的药物在琼脂中扩散，随着扩散距离的增加，抗菌药物的浓度呈对数减少，从而在纸片的周围形成浓度梯度。在纸片周围抑菌浓度范围内的细菌的生长被抑制，形成透明的抑菌环。抑菌环直径的大小可反映测试菌对测定药物的敏感程度，并与该药对测试菌的最低抑菌浓度（MIC）呈负相关，即抑菌环越大，越敏感，MIC 越小。

【实验器材】

（1）金黄色葡萄球菌、大肠杆菌 6~8h 肉汤培养物。

（2）普通琼脂平板。

（3）含各种抗菌药物的纸片（青霉素、链霉素、氯霉素、庆大霉素、先锋霉素、红霉素等）。

（4）酒精灯、接种环、小镊子、尺子、温箱等。

【实验方法】

（1）取琼脂平板两个，分别接种金黄色葡萄球菌和大肠杆菌，用平行划线法轻轻将菌液均匀地密涂于琼脂平板表面。用蜡笔将平板底均分为六部分，并标明六种抗生素及菌别。

（2）用无菌镊子取上述六种抗生素滤纸片，轻轻等距离贴于两个培养基的相应区域内，用镊子稍压，使之贴紧。底向上放于 37℃温箱中培养 18~24h 后，取出观察抑菌环直径的大小，以判定其敏感程度。

纸片扩散法如图 20 所示。

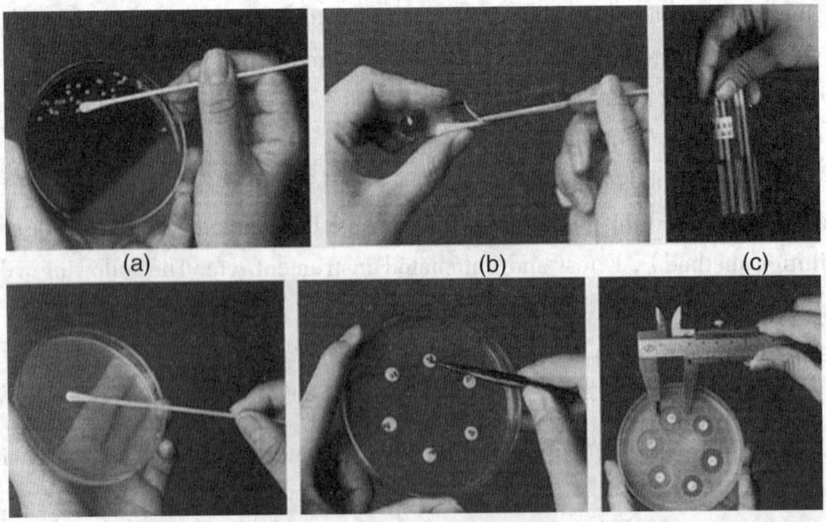

(a) (b) (c)

(d) (e) (f)

图 20 纸片扩散法

commonly used in clinical. The filter papers containing certain concentration of antimicrobial drugs are pasted on the surface of the agar plate which has been inoculated with testing bacteria, the drug will diffuse in agar. With the increasing diffusion distance, the concentration of antimicrobial drugs logarithmically reduces, forming a concentration gradient around the paper. The growth of bacteria within the bacteriostatic concentration around the paper is inhibited which causes a transparent bacterial inhibitory ring. The size of bacterial inhibitory ring can reflect the level of bacterial sensitivity to the drug. The drug sensitivity of bacteria has a reverse relationship with the minimal inhibitory concentration (MIC) of the drug, meaning that the larger the bacterial inhibitory ring, the more sensitive the bacteria to the drug and the smaller the MIC.

**【Materials and Equipment】**

(1) Broth cultures of *Staphylococcus aureus*, *Escherichia coli* which are cultured for 6–8h.

(2) Ordinary agar plate.

(3) Filter papers containing various kinds of antibacterial drugs (such as penicillin, streptomycin, chloramphenicol, gentamycin, cephalothin, erythromycin and so on).

(4) Alcohol lamp, inoculation loops, tweezers, rulers, thermostat, etc.

**【Methods】**

(1) Inoculate *Staphylococcus aureus* and *Escherichia coli* on the whole surface of two ordinary agar plates, respectively through parallel streak method. Divide the plate on the back into six parts and mark the six different kinds of antibiotics in each part.

(2) Paste the six kinds of drug containing filter papers on the corresponding and equal distance zone of the two plates with sterile tweezers. Press the papers gently with tweezers to make sure that they are tightly pasted. Incubate the plates in 37℃ thermostat for 18–24h and then observe the diameter of the bacteria inhibitory ring to determine the bacterial sensitivity.

Paper disk diffusion method is shown in Figure 20.

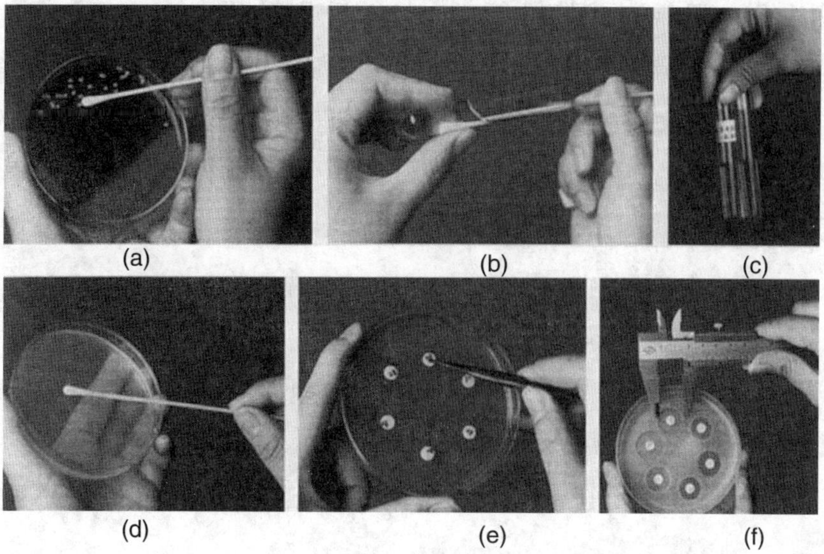

(a) (b) (c)

(d) (e) (f)

Figure 20 Paper Disk Diffusion Method

【实验结果】

细菌对药物敏感时，在该药纸片周围无细菌生长，形成抑菌环。细菌对药物不敏感，则药纸片周围有细菌生长。一般认为抑菌环直径 6~10mm 为低度敏感，10~15mm 为中度敏感，15mm 以上为高度敏感。

【思考题】

革兰阳细菌和阴性菌对各种抗生素的敏感性为什么不同?

（二）E 实验

【实验目的】

熟悉 E 实验的原理、操作方法和结果的判读。

【实验器材】

大肠杆菌琼脂平板培养物，MH 琼脂平板，E 试条。

【实验方法】

（1）菌液的准备：取培养 18~20h 的大肠杆菌菌落数个，均匀混悬于生理盐水中，调整其浓度至 0.5 麦氏比浊标准。

（2）接种：用无菌棉拭子蘸取菌液，在管内壁旋转挤去多余水分，均匀涂于琼脂平板表面。

（3）平板置室温或温箱 10~15min，让琼脂表面菌液吸收，以保证在加 E 试条前琼脂表面完全干燥。

（4）用无菌镊子将 E 试条贴于琼脂平板表面（E 试条 MIC 刻度面朝上，浓度最大端靠近平板边缘），置于 37℃温箱中孵育 16~20h 后观察结果。

【实验结果】

孵育后围绕试条形成一椭圆形的抑菌圈，抑菌圈与试条的交界处的刻度浓度即为抗菌药物对该细菌的 MIC 值。（见图 21）

【Results】

There is no growth around the paper when the bacterium is drug-sensitive, and this ring without bacterial growth is called bacterial inhibition ring. If the bacterium is not sensitive to the drug, there are many bacterial colonies around the paper. It is generally believed that it is low sensitivity when the diameter of bacteria inhibition ring is 6~10mm, moderate sensitive for 10–15mm, and high sensitive for larger than 15 mm.

【Questions】

Why the sensitivities to various antibiotics are different between Gram-positive bacteria and Gram-negative bacteria?

2. E Test

【Aim】

Get familiar with the principle, operation method and the result interpretation of E test.

【Materials and Equipment】

*Escherichia coli* cultured on agar plate, MH agar plate, E-strip.

【Methods】

(1) Preparation of bacterial solution: Take several *Escherichia coli* colonies that have been cultured for 18–20h and suspend in normal saline. Adjust the concentration of the solution to 0.5 McFarland Standard.

(2) Inoculation: Dip a sterile cotton swab in the *Escherichia coli* solution, remove excessive water and spread the bacteria on the surface of an agar plate.

(3) Incubate the plate at room temperature or in thermostat for 10–15min to let the bacterial solution absorbed on the agar surface to ensure that agar surface is completely dry before adding E-strip.

(4) Stick E-strip on the surface of the agar plate with a sterile tweezer(Be cautious that MIC scale of E-strip should be faced up and the pole with higher concentration is near the plate edges as well). Observe the result after putting it in 37℃ thermostat for 16–20h.

【Results】

There will be an oval bacterial inhibition ring around the strip after incubation. The number on the scale at the junction between the bacterial inhibition ring and the strip is the MIC value of the antimicrobial drug to the bacterium (Figure 21).

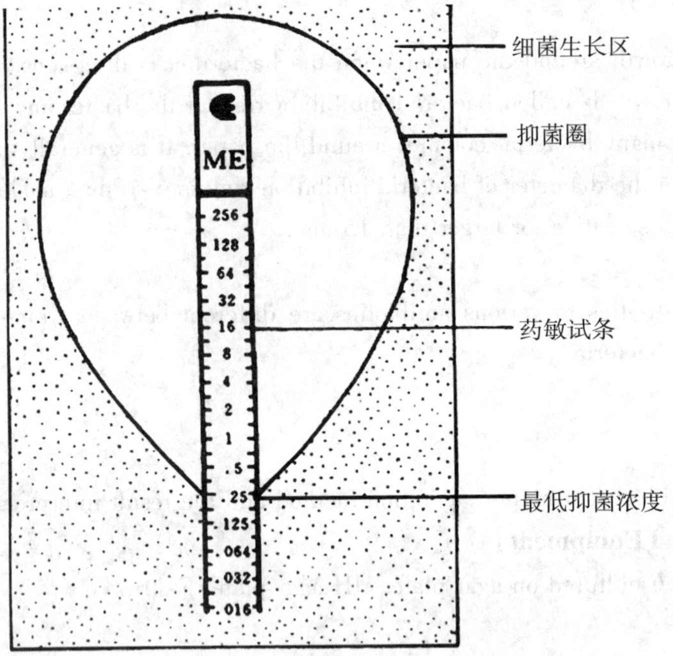


图 21　E 实验示意图

**【注意事项】**

(1) 药敏试条两侧的抑菌圈与 E 试条相交处介于 E 试条所示上下刻度之间时，读取较高的一侧所示的读数。

(2) 药敏试条两侧的抑菌圈与 E 试条相交处不一致时，读取刻度数值较高的一侧所示的读数。

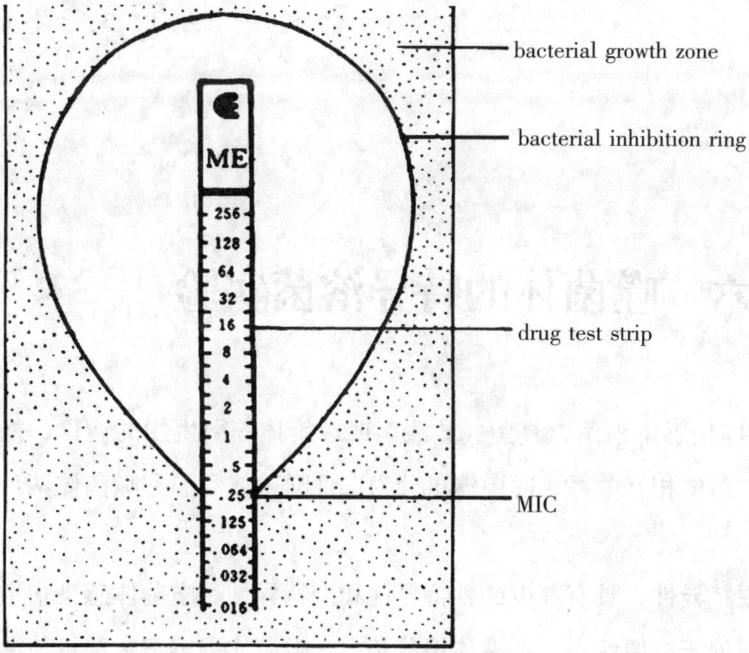


Figure 21 E test

**【Attentions】**

1. When the junctions between bacterial inhibition ring and E-strip locate between two calibrations of E-strip, the higher value should be taken.

2. When the junctions between bacterial inhibition ring and E-strip are at different scales of E-strip, the higher value should be taken.

# 实验十六　噬菌体的特异溶菌实验

噬菌体（bacteriophage）是感染细菌、真菌、放线菌或螺旋体等微生物的病毒，能通过细菌滤器。根据与宿主菌的相互关系，噬菌体可分为毒性噬菌体和温和噬菌体两种类型。

噬菌体具有严格的宿主特异性，具有高度的种特异性和型特异性。噬菌体感染宿主菌后，可裂解宿主细胞，或处于溶原状态。在液体培养基中，噬菌体裂解宿主菌可使混浊菌液变澄清；在固体培养基上，将适量的噬菌体和宿主菌液混合接种培养后，培养基表面可出现透亮的溶菌空斑，谓之噬斑。噬菌体可用于细菌的鉴定、分型，检查未知细菌等。

**【实验目的】**

掌握噬菌体对宿主感染的高度特异性。

**【实验器材】**

(1) 菌种：金黄色葡萄球菌及大肠杆菌纯培养物；大肠杆菌、痢疾杆菌和白色葡萄球菌肉汤培养物。

(2) 噬菌体：金黄色葡萄球菌噬菌体滤液、痢疾杆菌噬菌体滤液。

(3) 培养基：肉汤培养基、普通琼脂平板。

(4) 其他：无菌棉拭子、无菌吸管、温箱等。

**【实验方法】**

1. 液体培养基中噬菌体的溶菌现象

(1) 取 4 支肉汤管，2 支接种金黄色葡萄球菌，2 支接种大肠杆菌。

(2) 取上述两种细菌肉汤管各 1 支，分别加入金黄色葡萄球菌噬菌体滤液 0.2mL。

(3) 将上述 4 支肉汤管置于 37℃温箱中培养 6~12h 后观察结果。

2. 噬菌体的噬斑现象

(1) 取琼脂平板 1 个，将其分为 4 个等分区，注明①、②、③、④。

# XVI. The Specific Bacteriolytic Test of Bacteriophage

Bacteriophage is a kind of virus which can infect microorganisms such as bacteria, fungi, actinomyces or spirochaeta, and can pass through bacterial filters. They can be classified into virulent bacteriophage and temperate bacteriophage according to their relationship with the host bacteria.

Bacteriophage is of high host specificity and is species-specific and type-specific at the same time. Bacteriophage will either crack the host cells or be in the lysogenic state after infecting the host bacteria. It can make the cloudy bacterial solution become clear by cracking the host bacteria in the culture media. Inoculate and culture the mixture containing a proper dose of bacteriophage and host bacteria on the surface of a solid culture media, we can see bright lytic plaques on the surface. Bacteriophage can be used to identify, classify and check the unknown bacteria, etc.

**【Aim】**

To master the high specificity of bacteriophage when infecting the host.

**【Materials and Equipment】**

(1) Bacteria pure cultures of *Staphylococcus aureus* and *Escherichia coli*, broth cultures of *Escherichia coli*, *Bacillus dysenteriae* and *Staphylococcus albus*.

(2) Bacteriophage: bacteriophage filtrate of *Staphylococcus aureus*, bacteriophage filtrate of *Bacillus dysenteriae*.

(3) Medium: broth culture mediums, ordinary agar plates.

(4) Others: sterile cottor swabs, sterile pipette, thermostat.

**【Methods】**

### 1. The phenomenon of bacteriophage lysis in liquid medium

(1) Take 4 broth tubes. Inoculate two with *Staphylococcus aureus* and the other two with *Escherichia coli*.

(2) Take each one of those two kinds of bacteria broth tubes above, inject 0.2mL bacteriophage filtrate of *Staphylococcus aureus* into the tubes, respectively.

(3) Put the 4 broth tubes above in 37℃ thermostat for 6–12h, then observe the result.

### 2. Plaque phenomenon of bacteriophage

(1) Take an agar plate, divide it into 4 equal parts and mark with ①, ②, ③, ④.

(2) 分别用无菌棉拭子在①、②处涂布接种痢疾杆菌，在③处涂布接种大肠杆菌，在④处涂布接种白色葡萄球菌。

(3) 待涂布的菌液干后，在②、③、④处中央各加 1 小滴痢疾杆菌噬菌体滤液，在①处中央加 1 滴肉汤。

**【实验结果】**

(1) 液体培养基中噬菌体的溶菌现象：加有金黄色葡萄球菌噬菌体的金黄色葡萄球菌肉汤管变清，其余均混浊。

(2) 噬菌体的噬斑现象：在②处中央有一无菌生长的空斑，即噬斑，其余部位不出现噬斑。

(2) Inoculate bacteria evenly with sterile cotton swab over the plate, *Bacillus dysenteriae* over area ①, ②, *Escherichia coli* over area ③, *Staphylococcus albus* over area ④ .

(3) After coated bacteria solutions are dried, add a small drop of bacteriophage filtrate of *Bacillus dysenteriae* in the middle of area ②, ③, ④, and a drop of broth in the middle of area ①.

**【Results】**

(1) The phenomenon of bacteriophage lysis in liquid culture media: The *Staphylococcus aureus* broth tube added with bacteriophage of *Staphylococcus aureus* become clear and the rest of three tubes are turbid.

(2) Plaques phenomenon of bacteriophage: There is a sterile spot named plaque, which is in the middle of the area ②, and no plaques in other parts of the plate.

# 实验十七 病原菌的致病性实验

## 一、透明质酸酶的扩散作用

【实验原理】

透明质酸酶也称扩散因子。透明质酸是一种黏蛋白多糖，有高度的黏性，在结缔组织细胞间起“细胞黏合剂”的作用。细胞间的透明质酸被细菌产生的透明质酸酶分解后，细胞间隙扩大，通透性增加，细菌及其毒素易于向周围扩散。通过本实验可以观察透明质酸酶的侵袭作用。

【实验器材】

（1）家兔。

（2）溶血性链球菌24h肉汤培养物滤液。

（3）墨汁、生理盐水、70%酒精、无菌棉签等。

（4）无菌注射器、吸管、小试管、手术剪、镊子。

【实验方法】

（1）取家兔一只，剪去其背部两侧部分兔毛，用70%酒精局部消毒。

（2）用吸管吸取0.5mL溶血性链球菌培养物滤液，放入盛有0.5mL墨汁的小试管中，混匀。另取0.5mL生理盐水放入等量的墨汁小试管中充分混匀。

（3）在家兔背部两侧分别皮内注射两种混液各0.1mL（注射时要注意，勿使黑色素漏出），注入后立即量两侧黑色素扩散区直径，1h后再测两侧扩散区的直径，比较两侧记录结果。

【实验结果】

混有溶血性链球菌培养物滤液的黑色素扩散区明显大于生理盐水对照组扩散区。

## 二、血浆凝固酶实验

【实验目的】

掌握金黄色葡萄球菌的凝固酶实验原理及应用。

# XVII. Pathogenicity Test of Pathogenic Bacteria

## i . Diffusion Effect of Hyaluronidase

**【Principle】**

Hyaluronidase is also known as spreading factor. Hyaluronic acid is a glycosaminoglycan and has a high degree of viscosity which makes it the cell adherent reagent in connective tissues. If the hyaluronic acid among cells is decomposed by the hyaluronidase produced by the bacteria, the cell gap will be enlarged, the permeability will be increased, then the bacteria and toxins will be easier to spread. We can observe the invasion of hyaluronidase by this experiment.

**【Materials and Equipment】**

(1) Rabbits.

(2) Broth culture filtrate of *Streptococcus hemolyticus* (24h).

(3) Ink, normal saline, 70% alcohol, sterile cotton swab, etc.

(4) Sterile syringes, straws, small test tubes, operation scissors and tweezers.

**【Methods】**

(1) Take a rabbit, cut off the hair on both sides of its back. Disinfect with 70% alcohol.

(2) Take a small test tube which contains 0.5mL ink, add 0.5mL broth culture filtrate of *Streptococcus hemolyticus* and mix. Take another small test tube which contains 0.5mL ink, add 0.5mL normal saline and mix.

(3) Inject intradermally 0.1mL each kind of the mixed liquid in each side of the back skin of rabbit, respectively (Don't make the leakage of the black dye). After the injection, measure the diameter of the black dye diffusion area immediately and 1h after. Compare the results of both sides.

**【Results】**

The diameter of the black dye diffusion of *Streptococcus hemolyticus* group is significantly larger than that of normal saline.

## ii . Plasma Coagulase Test

**【Aim】**

To master the principle and application of the *Staphylococcus aureus* coagulase test.

【实验原理】

凝固酶实验是实验室鉴定葡萄球菌致病性的重要实验。致病性葡萄球菌可产生两种凝固酶，一种是与细胞壁结合的凝聚因子，称为结合凝固酶，它直接作用于血浆中的纤维蛋白质，使其发生沉淀，于细菌外面凝聚成块；另一种凝固酶分泌至菌体外，成为游离凝固酶，它能使纤维蛋白原变为纤维蛋白，从而使血浆凝固。血浆凝固酶实验被广泛用于常规鉴定金黄色葡萄球菌与其他葡萄球菌，常作为鉴定葡萄球菌致病性的主要依据之一。金黄色葡萄球菌的凝固酶为阳性，非致病性菌一般不产生此酶，因此，血浆凝固酶实验是鉴别葡萄球菌有无致病性的重要指标。

【实验器材】

(1) 金黄色葡萄球菌和表皮葡萄球菌血琼脂平板培养物。

(2) 抗凝兔血浆、生理盐水、毛细滴管、接种环、载玻片等。

【实验方法】

(1) 取洁净载玻片一张，于两端各加生理盐水一滴。

(2) 以灭菌接种环自血琼脂平板上挑取两种葡萄球菌培养物少许，分别混悬于玻片上的生理盐水内，使之呈均匀的细菌悬液，观察有无自凝现象，于每滴细菌悬液内，各加入抗凝兔血浆一滴，混匀。

(3) 数秒钟后观察结果，若细菌呈颗粒状凝集则为阳性，若无凝集则为阴性。

【实验结果】

金黄色葡萄球菌能产生血浆凝固酶，故为阳性；表皮葡萄球菌不能产生血浆凝固酶，故为阴性。

## 三、内毒素测定与鲎实验

【实验原理】

鲎实验是检测内毒素的一种实验方法，实验灵敏，能检出微量（0.000 1μg/mL）内毒素。鲎是一种冷血动物，其血细胞的溶解产物与内毒素相遇即被凝固，机制尚不清楚，可能是溶解物中含有凝固蛋白原和一种高相对分子质量的凝固酶原，凝固酶原经内毒素激活转化成凝固酶，此酶使蛋白酶原变为凝固蛋白，再通过交联酶的作用，相互聚合，形成纤维状凝胶。

【实验器材】

(1) 鲎实验试剂一套。

(2) 大肠杆菌内毒素（阳性对照）、无菌蒸馏水、待检液等。

**【Principle】**

Coagulase test is an important method to identify the pathogenicity of *Staphylococcus*. Pathogenic *Staphylococcus* can produce two types of coagulase: bound coagulase and free coagulase. While bound coagulase is a cell wall associated clumping factor which attaches to fiber protein directly and aggregates oustside the bacteria, free coagulase is an enzyme secreted extracellularly, which converts fibrinogen to fibrin resulting in clotting of plasma. Coagulase test is used widely in differentiating *Staphylococcus aureus* from other *Staphylococcus*, and is one of the main basis in identifying the pathogenicity of *Staphylococcus*. The coagulase of *Staphylococcus aureus* is positive, while non-pathogenic bacteria do not have this kind of coagulase, so plasma coagulase test is the most importarnt index in identifying the pathogenicity of *Staphylococcus*.

**【Materials and Equipment】**

(1) Blood agar plate culture of *Staphylococcus aureus* and *Staphylococcus epidermidis*.

(2) Rabbit anticoagulant plasma, normal saline, capillary burette, inoculation loop, slides, etc.

**【Methods】**

(1) Add one drop of normal saline on two ends of a clean slide.

(2) The two normal saline drops are emulsified with cultures of *Staphylococcus aureus* and *Staphylococcus epidermidis* by using sterile inoculation loops, respectively. Observe whether there is the apperance of self-clotting. A drop of plasma is then added into both mixtures and mix well, respectively.

(3) Observe the result after several seconds. It is positive if macroscopic clumping can be observed in the plasma and a negative reaction is indicated by no visible clumping.

**【Results】**

*Staphylococcus aureus* can produce coagulase and is coagulase-positive, while *Staphylococcus epidermidis* can't produce coagulase and is coagulase-negative.

## iii. Detection of Endotoxin and Limulus Test

**【Principle】**

Limulus test is a sensitive method used to test the presence of bacterial endotoxin, can detect micro-endotoxin (0.000,1μg/mL). Limulus is a kind of poikilotherm, and coagulation will occur if its blood cell lysate interacts with endotoxin. How the phenomenon happens is still not understood. It is speculated that the lysate contains coagulagen and a high molecular mass proclotting enzyme. This proclotting enzyme can be activated into coagulase by endotoxin, and the coagulase converts the coagulagen to coagulation protein, forming fibrillar gels through the role of cross-linked enzyme and mutual polymerization.

**【Materials and Equipment】**

(1) A set of limulus reagent.

(2) *Escherichia coli* endotoxin (positive control), sterile distilled water, sample to be detected.

(3) 吸管、小试管、试管架等。

【实验方法】

(1) 将鲎实验试剂按要求加入等量的不含有热原质的无菌蒸馏水，振摇 2~3min 使之溶解。

(2) 在实验管、阳性对照管及空白对照管中各加溶解物 0.1mL。

(3) 在实验管中加待检液 0.1mL，阳性对照管加大肠杆菌内毒素 0.1mL，空白对照管加蒸馏水 0.1mL，37℃水浴 1h 后观察结果。结果如表 1 所示。

表 1 鲎实验

| | 实验管 | 阳性对照管 | 空白对照管 |
|---|---|---|---|
| 鲎试剂溶解物（mL） | 0.1 | 0.1 | 0.1 |
| 待检样品（mL） | 0.1 | — | — |
| 大肠杆菌内毒素（mL） | — | 0.1 | — |
| 蒸馏水（mL） | — | — | 0.1 |
| 37℃水浴 1h 后观察结果 | 凝固 | 凝固 | 未凝固 |

【实验结果】

(1) 阳性对照管出现凝固，空白对照管无变化时，实验结果正确，再观察实验管。

(2) 实验管出现凝固为阳性，证明有内毒素存在，如未出现凝固，则证明无内毒素存在。

(3) Straw, small test tube, test tube rack, etc.

**【Methods】**

(1) Add equal amount of sterile distilled water which does not contain pyrogen to the limulus reagent according to the requirements, shake 2–3min to dissolve it.

(2) Add 0.1mL limulus reagent fluid to the detection tube, the positive control tube and the blank control tube, respectively.

(3) Add 0.1mL sample to be detected to the detection tube, 0.1mL *Escherichia coli* endotoxin to the positive control tube and 0.1mL sterile distilled water to the blank control tube. Observe the result after 1h at 37℃ water bath. The result is shown in Table 1.

Table 1 Limulus Test

| | detection tube | positive control tube | blank control tube |
|---|---|---|---|
| limulus reagent fluid (mL) | 0.1 | 0.1 | 0.1 |
| sample to be detected (mL) | 0. 1 | — | — |
| *Escherichia coli* endotoxin (mL) | — | 0.1 | — |
| sterile distilled water (mL) | — | — | 0.1 |
| observe after 1h at 37℃ water bath | | | |
| results | coagulation | coagulation | no coagulation |

**【Results】**

(1) If coagulation occurs in positive control tube and dosen't occur in the blank control tube, the result is correct and we can observe the detection tube.

(2) The coagulation indicates the presence of endotoxin, if there is no coagulation, then there is no endotoxin.

# 实验十八　溶菌酶实验

溶菌酶是一种碱性蛋白质，广泛分布于血清、泪液、唾液及鼻腔分泌物中，主要作用于革兰阳性菌。测定体液和分泌物中溶菌酶的含量及其变动情况，可作为了解机体天然抵抗力的指标之一，测定方法有分光光度计测定法和琼脂平板测定法。

**【实验原理】**

溶菌酶作用于革兰阳性菌细胞壁的肽聚糖，使之分解，令细胞壁失去韧性，使细菌发生渗透性溶解。通过本实验可以了解溶菌酶的杀菌原理，观察溶菌现象。

**【实验器材】**

（1）菌种：溶壁微球菌（*M. lysodeikticus*）菌液。

（2）培养基：1%高层琼脂。

（3）无菌平皿、恒温水浴箱、打孔器、毛细吸管等。

**【实验方法】**

**琼脂平板测定法**

（1）溶壁微球菌菌液 1mL 加入无菌平皿中，然后加入融化的高层琼脂（冷至 60~70℃）15mL 混匀，厚约 4mm，静置待凝。

（2）用打孔器打四个孔，距离相等。

（3）用毛细吸管于三个孔中各加唾液至满，另一孔加生理盐水作为对照。

（4）置于 24~26℃恒温水浴箱中孵育 15~18h，观察孔周围的溶菌环并测其直径大小。

**【实验结果】**

唾液中含溶菌酶，使溶壁微球菌溶解，孔周围出现透明的无菌环，环的直径与溶菌酶的浓度成正比，生理盐水对照孔周围无溶菌环出现。

# XVIII. Lysozyme Test

Lysozyme, a kind of alkaline protein, is abundant in serum, tears, saliva, and nasal secretions, and mainly affects Gram-positive bacteria. The level of lysozyme in body fluids and secretions and its change can be used as an indicator to understand the natural resistance of the body. Spectrophotometric determination method and agar plate method can be used.

**【Principle】**

The lysozyme attacks the peptidoglycan of the cell wall of Gram-positive bacteria, making the cell wall loss resilience and osmotic dissolution occurs. In this experiment, we can observe the bacteriolytic phenomenon and understand the principle of the bactericidal action by lysozyme.

**【Materials and Equipment】**

(1) Bacteria: *M. lysodeikticus* bacterial solution.

(2) Culture medium: 1% top agar .

(3) Sterile plate, thermostatic water bath, puncher, capillary straw, etc.

**【Methods】**

### Agar plate method

(1) Add 1mL *M. lysodeikticus* to the sterile plate, and then add 15mL melting top agar (60–70℃) and mix. The thickness is about 4mm. Wait until it is solidified.

(2) Punch four wells on the plate by puncher and make sure the distance is equal.

(3) Fill three of the wells with saliva and fill another well with normal saline as control.

(4) Culture the plate in thermostatic water bath at 24–26℃ for 15–18h, and then observe the bacteriolytic ring and measure its diameter.

**【Results】**

The lysozyme of saliva dissolves the *M. lysodeikticus*. Transparent rings appear around the wells, and the diameter of the ring is proportional to the lysozyme concentration. There is no bacteriolytic ring in control well.

# 实验十九 病原性球菌

病原性球菌主要包括葡萄球菌、链球菌、肺炎球菌、脑膜炎球菌及淋球菌，是常见的人类化脓性感染病原体，故又称为化脓性球菌。

## 一、葡萄球菌、链球菌、肺炎球菌、脑膜炎球菌和淋球菌的形态及染色性

**【实验原理】**

葡萄球菌、链球菌、肺炎球菌、脑膜炎球菌和淋球菌的形态及染色特点各不相同。

**【实验器材】**

（1）金黄色葡萄球菌、链球菌、肺炎球菌、脑膜炎球菌及淋球菌革兰染色标本片。

（2）肺炎球菌荚膜染色标本片。

（3）普通光学显微镜、镜油、擦镜纸等。

**【实验方法】**

在普通光学显微镜上观察上述病原性球菌。

**【实验结果】**

（1）金黄色葡萄球菌菌体呈球形，排列成葡萄串状，革兰染色阳性。

（2）链球菌菌体呈球形或卵圆形，链状排列，革兰染色阳性。

（3）肺炎球菌菌体呈卵圆形或矛头状，常成双排列，钝端相对，尖端相背。菌体外有明显荚膜，革兰染色阳性。在普通染色标本中，因荚膜不易着色，在荚膜区呈现不着色的半透明环，围绕在菌体外面。用特殊染色（荚膜染色）法可使荚膜着色。本次观察标本使用赫斯荚膜染色法，菌体与背景均呈紫色，荚膜为淡蓝色。

（4）在患者脑脊液涂片标本中，脑膜炎球菌常位于中性粒细胞内外，菌体呈肾形，成双排列，凹面相对，革兰染色阴性。

（5）淋球菌常成双排列，两球菌的接触面平坦，染色标本中形似一对咖啡豆，革兰染色阴性。

# XIX. Pathogenic Cocci

Pathogenic cocci include *Staphylococcus, Streptococcus, Streptococcus pneumoniae, Neisseria meningitidis and Gonococcus*, which are common pathogen in human pyogenic infection, so they are also called pyogenic cocci.

## i . The Morphology and Staining Characteristics of *Staphylococcus, Streptococcus, Streptococcus Pneumoniae, Neisseria Meningitidis* and *Gonococcus*

**【Principle】**

The morphology and staining characteristics of *Staphylococcus, Streptococcus, Streptococcus pneumoniae, Neisseria meningitidis* and *Gonococcus* are different from each other.

**【Materials and Equipment】**

(1) *Staphylococcus aureus* Gram-stained smears, *Streptococcus* Gram-stained smears, *Streptococcus pneumoniae* Gram-stained smears, *Neisseria meningitidis* Gram-stained smears and *Gonococcus* Gram-stained smears.

(2) *Streptococcus pneumoniae* capsule staining smears.

(3) Ordinary optical microscope, immersion oil, lens paper, etc.

**【Methods】**

Observe the above pathogenic cocci with ordinary optical microscope.

**【Results】**

(1) *Staphylococcus aureus* is spherical and Gram-positive, and arranges in thyrsiform.

(2) *Streptococcus* is spherical or oval and Gram-positive, and arranges in chains.

(3) *Streptococcus pneumoniae* is in oval or spear shape, and Gram-positive, often arranges in pairs, the blunt end toward the blunt end. There are obvious capsules outside the bacterial body, which are not easy to be colored and appear uncolored translucent ring outside around the bacterial body in ordinary stained specimens. The capsule can be colored with special staining (capsule staining) method. The specimen in this observation is made by Hiss's capsule staining method in which the bacterial bodies and the background appear purple, and the capsules are stained light blue.

(4) In smears made by cerebrospinal fluid from patients, we can observe *Neisseria meningitidis* in or outside the neutrophils. They are in kidney shape and Gram-negative, arrange in pairs, the concave toward the concave.

## 二、葡萄球菌、链球菌及肺炎球菌培养特性

【实验原理】

金黄色葡萄球菌、表皮葡萄球菌、腐生葡萄球菌、甲型溶血性链球菌、乙型溶血性链球菌及肺炎球菌在血琼脂平板上的菌落特点及溶血性各不相同。

【实验器材】

金黄色葡萄球菌、表皮葡萄球菌、腐生葡萄球菌、甲型溶血性链球菌、乙型溶血性链球菌及肺炎球菌血琼脂平板培养物。

【实验方法】

观察上述细菌的血琼脂平板培养物，比较每种菌单个菌落的形态、大小、表面、边缘、透明度、颜色及溶血性。

【实验结果】

(1) 三种葡萄球菌在普通琼脂平板上形成中等大小、圆形、表面光滑、边缘整齐、不透明的菌落，并可产生不同的脂溶性色素，金黄色葡萄球菌产生金黄色色素，表皮葡萄球菌大多产生白色色素，腐生葡萄球菌大多产生柠檬色色素。三种葡萄球菌在血琼脂平板上出现的菌落类似它们在普通琼脂平板上的菌落，但金黄色葡萄球菌菌落周围有明显的溶血环，而表皮葡萄球菌和腐生葡萄球菌菌落周围无溶血环。

(2) 链球菌在血琼脂平板上生长后出现灰白色针尖大小菌落，菌落周围可出现不同的溶血情况，甲型链球菌菌落周围出现草绿色溶血环，乙型链球菌菌落周围出现透明溶血环。

(3) 肺炎球菌在血琼脂平板上形成圆形、光滑、扁平、透明或半透明的细小菌落。在菌落周围有草绿色狭窄溶血环，与甲型链球菌相似。培养时间稍久，因本菌产生自溶酶，出现自溶现象，致使菌落中央凹陷，呈脐状。

## 三、抗链球菌溶血素 O（ASO）的检测

【实验原理】

本试剂胶乳液是由溶血素“O”和羧化聚苯乙烯胶乳共价交联而成的抗原胶乳。将 ASO 胶乳的灵敏度调整到 200IU/mL，超过上述滴度即出现肉眼可见凝集颗粒，使用本试剂血清标本不需要稀释即可直接测定。

【实验器材】

(1) 胶乳液成分：链球菌溶血素“O”胶乳、牛血清白蛋白、磷酸盐缓冲液。

(2) 阳性对照成分：羊抗 SLO 抗血清、牛血清白蛋白、磷酸盐缓冲液。

(5) Gonococcus are Gram-negative, often arrange in pairs. The contact surface of two bacterial body is always flat and that makes them look like coffee beans.

## ii . The Culture Characteristics of *Staphylococcus, Streptococcus* and *Streptococcus Pneumoniae*

**【Principle】**

The colony and hemolysis characteristics of *Staphylococcus aureus, Staphylococcus epidermidis, Staphylococcus saprophyticus, α-hemolytic Streptococcus* and *β-hemolytic Streptococcus,* and *Streptococcus pneumoniae* are different from each other on the blood agar plates.

**【Materials and Equipment】**

The cultures of *Staphylococcus aureus, Staphylococcus epidermidis, Staphylococcus saprophyticus, α-hemolytic Streptococcus* and *β-hemolytic Streptococcus*, and *Streptococcus pneumoniae* on blood agar plates.

**【Methods】**

Observe the cultures and compare the colony morphology, size, surface, edge, transparency, color, and hemolysis of each kind of bacteria.

**【Results】**

(1) Three kinds of *Staphylococci* form medium-sized, round, smooth surfaced, smooth edged, and opaque colonies on the ordinary agar plates, producing a variety of lipid-soluble pigments. *Staphylococcus aureus* produces yellow pigment, *Staphylococcus epidermidis* always produces white pigment, *Staphylococcus saprophyticus* produces lemon pigment. On the blood agar plates, the colonies of the three species are similar, but there are marked hemolytic rings around *Staphylococcus aureus* colonies and none around *Staphylococcus epidermidis* colonies and *Staphylococcus saprophyticus* colonies.

(2) The *Streptococcus* forms pale white colonies in tip size on the blood agar plate, and different hemolytic situations appear around the colonies. There are grass green hemolytic rings around *α-hemolytic Streptococcus* colonies, and transparent hemolytic rings around *β-hemolytic Streptococcus* colonies.

(3) The *Streptococcus pneumoniae* forms round, smooth, flat, transparent or semi-transparent small colonies on the blood agar plates. Like *α-hemolytic Streptococcus*, they form grass green narrow hemolytic rings. When the incubation time is prolonged, the bacteria appear autolysis due to the autolysis enzyme produced by themself, forming an umbilical shape with central depression in the colony.

## iii . Anti-Streptolysin O (ASO) Detection

**【Principle】**

This reagent is an antigen latex containing hemolysin "O" covalently cross-linked on carboxylated polystyrene latex. ASO sensitivity is adjusted to 200IU/mL, above which visible agglutination particles appear in samples. When using this reagent, serum samples can be detected directly without the need of dilution.

(3) 阴性对照成分：牛血清白蛋白、磷酸盐缓冲液。

(4) 患者血清。

(5) 微量反应板、微量加样器及吸头等。

**【实验方法】**

1. 定性实验

试剂使用前，预置达室温；轻轻混匀胶乳试剂；核对阴性和阳性对照；在反应板孔中加一滴未稀释血清（50μL）；然后在血清中加一滴胶乳试剂，搅匀、轻轻摇动使其充分混合，两分钟后观察结果。阴性和阳性对照同上法操作。

2. 半定量实验

血清以生理盐水（0.9g 氯化钠溶解于蒸馏水中，稀释至 100mL）倍比稀释，可参照上法操作。

正常参考范围：0~200IU/mL。

检验结果分析：凝集出现可判断样本中 ASO>200IU/mL，阳性；无凝集出现可判断样本中 ASO<200IU/mL，阴性。

**【注意事项】**

(1) 加试剂时，应保证液滴大小一致。

(2) 若阴性、阳性对照结果出现异常，则试剂不可使用。

(3) 试剂盒贮存于 2~10℃，受热会导致试剂阳性率偏高，切勿冷冻。

(4) 阴性、阳性对照经检测 HbsAg、HCV、HIV 为阴性，但仍须如病人样品一样小心。

**【Materials and Equipment】**

(1) The ingredients of latex: streptolysin "O" latex, bovine serum albumin, phosphate buffer.

(2) The ingredients of positive control: Sheep anti-SLO serum, bovine serum albumin, phosphate buffer.

(3) The ingredients of negative control: bovine serum albumin, phosphate buffer.

(4) Patient serum.

(5) The micro reaction plate, micropipettes and tips.

**【Procedures】**

### 1. Qualitative experiment

Reagent should be preset up to room temperature before use; gently mix latex reagent; check the negative and positive controls; add one drop of undiluted serum (50μL) in the reaction well of the plate; then add a drop of latex reagent in the serum; stir gently to make it fully mixed, observe after two minutes. Perform same procedures with negative and positive controls.

### 2. Semi-quantitative experiment

Serum is diluted with normal saline (0.9g sodium chloride dissolved in 100mL distilled water) in series, and perform the above operation.

Reference value: 0–200IU/mL)

Test results analysis: agglutination indicates ASO titer in samples is above 200IU/mL, no agglutination indicates ASO titer is below 200IU/mL.

**【Attentions】**

(1) Ensure the droplet size consistent when adding reagent.

(2) If the result of positive or negative control is abnormal, the reagent should not be used.

(3) Store the kit at 2–10 degree, heating will lead to higher positive rate. Do not freeze the kit.

(4) Even the negative and positive controls are detected as HbsAg, HCV and HIV negative, caution should still be paid same as patient samples.

# 实验二十 肠道杆菌

【实验目的】

(1) 掌握肠道杆菌的形态及染色性、培养特性。

(2) 掌握肠道杆菌生化反应的原理和方法。

(3) 掌握肠道杆菌生化反应的鉴别。

【实验原理】

肠道杆菌是一大群生物学性状相似的革兰阴性无芽胞杆菌，大多数寄生在人和动物的肠道中，也存在于水、土壤或腐败的物质上，有的构成肠道正常菌群，如大肠杆菌等；有的经消化道侵入后，对人类有明显的致病作用，如沙门菌、痢疾杆菌等。

一般用生化反应初步鉴定肠道杆菌，然后依据各菌的抗原特异性进一步作血清学鉴定。

## 一、肠道杆菌的形态及染色性

【实验器材】

(1) 大肠杆菌，伤寒杆菌，甲、乙型副伤寒杆菌及福氏、宋内痢疾杆菌革兰染色标本片。

(2) 普通光学显微镜、镜油、擦镜纸。

【实验方法】

取上述肠道杆菌革兰染色标本片置显微镜下，观察细菌形态及染色特点。

【实验结果】

上述肠道杆菌均为革兰阴性短杆菌，形态染色不易区别。

## 二、肠道杆菌培养特性

【实验器材】

大肠杆菌，伤寒杆菌，甲、乙型副伤寒杆菌及福氏、宋内痢疾杆菌 SS 琼脂平板培养物。

# XX. *Enterobacteriaceae*

**【Aim】**

(1) To master the morphology and staining characteristics, culture characteristics of *Enterobacteriaceae*.

(2) To master the principles and methods of biochemical reaction of *Enterobacteriaceae*.

(3) To master the identification of the biochemical reaction of *Enterobacteriaceae*.

**【Principle】**

*Enterobacteriaceae* is a large group of non-spore Gram-negative bacilli which have the similar biological characteristics. Most of them not only parasitize in the intestines of humans and animals, but also exist in the water, soil and decomposing things. Some constitute the normal intestinal flora, such as *Escherichia coli*. Some have obvious pathogenic effects on humans by invading through intestines, such as *Salmonella*, *Bacillus dysenteriae* and so on.

Identification of *Enterobacteriaceae* generally makes preliminary identification with biochemical reactions. And then further serologic identification can be made on the basis of the antigen specificity.

## i. The Morphology and Staining Characteristics of *Enterobacteriaceae*

**【Materials and Equipment】**

(1) Gram-stained smears of *Escherichia coli*, *Salmonella typhi*, *Salmonella paratyphi A*, *Salmonella paratyphi B* and *Shigella flexneri*, *Shigella sonnei*.

(2) Ordinary optical microscope, immersion oil, lens paper.

**【Methods】**

Put the above Gram-stained smears of *Enterobacteriaceae* under the microscope to observe the morphology and staining characteristics of bacteria.

**【Results】**

All of these bacteria are Gram-negative bacillus brevis, which are not easy to distinguish.

## ii. Culture Characteristics of *Enterobacteriaceae*

**【Materials and Equipment】**

SS agar plate cultures of *Escherichia coli*, *Salmonella typhi*, *Salmonella paratyphi A*, *Salmonella paratyphi B* and *Shigella flexneri*, *Shigella sonnei*.

【实验方法】

分别观察大肠杆菌，伤寒杆菌，甲、乙型副伤寒杆菌，福氏、宋内痢疾杆菌在SS琼脂平板上生长的菌落，注意其大小、颜色及透明度。

【实验结果】

(1) 大肠杆菌菌落较大，光滑湿润，不透明，在琼脂平板上形成蓝色菌落，在SS琼脂平板上形成红色菌落。

(2) 三种沙门菌均形成无色、半透明、中等大小的菌落。

(3) 两种痢疾杆菌菌落与沙门菌菌落相似。

## 三、肠道杆菌的生化反应

【实验器材】

(1) 大肠杆菌，伤寒杆菌，甲、乙型副伤寒杆菌，福氏痢疾杆菌，普通变形杆菌六种肠道杆菌生化反应管（葡萄糖、乳糖、甘露糖、靛基质、硫化氢、尿素分解和动力实验）培养物。

(2) 上述六种肠道杆菌蛋白胨水培养物。

【实验方法】

(1) 观察上述六种肠道杆菌的生长情况，注意有无动力和颜色变化。

(2) 观察上述六种肠道杆菌在单糖发酵管内的生长情况，注意是否产酸、产气。

(3) 于上述六种肠道杆菌蛋白胨水培养物内，分别加入靛基质（吲哚）试剂，观察有无吲哚产生。

【实验结果】

六种肠道杆菌生化反应结果见下表（表2）：

**表2 六种肠道杆菌生化反应结果**

| 菌名 | 葡萄糖 | 甘露醇 | 乳糖 | 靛基质 | 硫化氢 | 尿素分解 | 动力 |
|---|---|---|---|---|---|---|---|
| 大肠杆菌 | ⊕ | ⊕ | ⊕ | + | – | – | + |
| 伤寒杆菌 | + | + | – | – | –/+ | – | + |
| 甲型副伤寒杆菌 | ⊕ | ⊕ | – | – | –/+ | – | + |
| 乙型副伤寒杆菌 | ⊕ | ⊕ | – | – | + | – | + |
| 福氏痢疾杆菌 | + | + | – | –/+ | – | – | – |
| 普通变形杆菌 | ⊕ | – | – | + | + | + | + |

注: +表示产酸或阳性，⊕表示产酸和产气，–表示无变化或阴性。

【Methods】

Observe the colonies of *Escherichia coli, Salmonella typhi, Salmonella paratyphi A, Salmonella paratyphi B, Shigella flexneri, Shigella sonnei* on SS agar plate, respectively. Pay attention to the size, color and transparency.

【Results】

(1) The colony of *Escherichia coli* is big, smooth, moist and not transparent. It is blue on the agar plate but red on the SS agar plate.

(2) The colonies of the three types of *Salmonella* are colorless, transparent, medium size.

(3) The colonies of the two types of *Bacillus dysenteriae* are similar to that of *Salmonella.*

## ⅲ. Biochemical Reactions of *Enterobacteriaceae*

【Materials and Equipment】

(1) Biochemical reaction tube cultures of *Escherichia coli, Salmonella typhi, Salmonella paratyphi A, Salmonella paratyphi B, Shigella flexneri, Bacillus proteus* (glucose, lactose, mannose, indole, hydrogen sulfide, urea decomposition and dynamic experiment).

(2) Peptone water cultures of the above six kinds of *Enterobacteriaceae.*

【Methods】

(1) Observe the growth of the above six kinds of *Enterobacteriaceae.* Pay attention to the presence of power and the color change.

(2) Observe the growth of the above six kinds of *Enterobacteriaceae* in fermentation tube. Pay attention to that if any acid or gas is produced.

(3) Add indole reagent into peptone water cultures of these six kinds of *Enterobacteriaceae* respectively and observe the presence of indole.

【Results】

The results of biochemical reaction of these six kinds of *Enterobacteriaceae* are shown in the table below (Table 2):

Table 2 The Results of Biochemical Reaction of Six Kinds of *Enterobacteriaceae*

| bacteria name | glucose | lactose | mannose | indole | hydrogen sulfide | urea decomposition | dynamics |
|---|---|---|---|---|---|---|---|
| *Escherichia coli* | ⊕ | ⊕ | ⊕ | + | − | − | + |
| *Salmonella typhi* | + | + | − | − | −/+ | − | + |
| *Salmonella paratyphi A* | ⊕ | ⊕ | − | − | −/+ | − | + |
| *Salmonella paratyphi B* | ⊕ | ⊕ | − | − | + | − | + |
| *Shigella flexneri* | + | + | − | −/+ | − | − | − |
| *Bacillus proteus* | ⊕ | − | − | + | + | + | + |

Note: + indicates acid production or positive, ⊕indicates the production of acid and gas, − indicates no change or negative.

**【思考题】**

(1) 肠道杆菌有什么共同特征?

(2) 如何鉴别致病性肠道杆菌?

**【Questions】**

(1) What are the common characteristics of *Enterobacteriaceae*?

(2) How to identify pathogenic *Enterobacteriaceae*?

# 实验二十一 粪便标本中致病性肠道杆菌的分离与鉴定

**【实验目的】**

通过本实验初步掌握从粪便标本中分离与鉴定致病性肠道杆菌的方法。

**【实验原理】**

致病性肠道杆菌主要有伤寒杆菌、副伤寒杆菌和痢疾杆菌等，它们都是革兰阴性杆菌，在形态上相互间不易鉴别。肠道正常菌群中的大肠杆菌也是革兰阴性杆菌，在形态上与致病性肠道杆菌难以区别。欲从粪便标本中检出致病性肠道杆菌，达到对传染病进行病原学诊断的目的，必须首先把粪便中的肠道杆菌各自分开，再依其生化反应、血清学实验进行鉴定。

SS 培养基为分离肠道病原菌的选择培养基。中性红在培养基中起指示剂作用，大肠杆菌能迅速分解乳糖产酸，并与胆盐结合成胆酸，故菌落是粉红色；病原菌不分解乳糖，故菌落为微黄色或无色。培养基中的胆盐、枸橼酸盐对革兰阳性杆菌及多数大肠杆菌有较强的抑制作用。硫代硫酸钠有缓和胆盐对志贺菌及沙门菌的毒性作用，并中和煌绿、中性红染剂的毒性。

半固体双糖含铁培养基以酚红为指示剂，酸性时呈黄色，碱性时呈红色。下层为含葡萄糖的半固体培养基，可以观察细菌的动力和对葡萄糖的发酵能力。上层为含乳糖的亚铁固体，主要观察细菌对乳糖的发酵情况，产生 $H_2S$ 的能力。葡萄糖含量仅为乳糖的 1/10，若细菌只分解葡萄糖，不分解乳糖，则产酸量少，斜面部分因接触空气而氧化，所以斜面和底层先呈黄色，后来斜面变成红色。若细菌分解双糖而产酸产气，则培养基均呈黄色，且有气泡产生。细菌产生 $H_2S$ 时，遇硫酸亚铁，形成黑色硫化铁。

**【实验器材】**

(1) 病人粪便标本。

(2) SS 琼脂平板、半固体双糖含铁培养基、沙门菌与痢疾杆菌诊断血清等。

# XXI. The Separation and Identification of Pathogenic *Enterobacteriaceae* in Feces Specimens

【Aim】

To initially master the method of the separation and identification of pathogenic *Enterobacteriaceae* in feces specimens.

【Principle】

Pathogenic *Enterobacteriaceae* mainly includes *Salmonella typhi*, *Salmonella paratyphi* and *Bacillus dysenteriae*, which are Gram-negative bacilli, and difficult to distinguish from their morphological differences. *Escherichia coli* in normal intestinal flora is Gram-negative bacteria, which is also difficult to differentiate from pathogenic *Enterobacteriaceae* in shape. For detection of pathogenic *Enterobacteriaceae* in feces specimens and etiological diagnosis of infectious diseases, we must firstly isolate different *Enterobacteriaceae* from feces specimens and then identify them on the basis of their biochemical and serological tests.

SS medium is a selective medium that separates intestinal pathogens. Neutral red is an indicator in the medium, and *Escherichia coli* quickly break down lactose to produce acid and bind cholate to produce cholic acid, so the colony is pink. Pathogens don't break down lactose, and get the slightly yellow or colorless colonies. Cholate, citrate in medium can inhibit Gram-positive bacteria and most of *Escherichia coli*. $Na_2S_2O_3$ weakens toxic effects of cholate on *Shigella* and *Salmonella* , and neutralizes the toxicity of brilliant green and neutral red dye.

Phenol red is an indicator of semi-solid disaccharide iron medium. When the medium is acidic, phenol red changes into yellow; when alkaline, phenol red changes into red. In semi-solid medium, the lower part contains glucose and bacteria's movement and ability to ferment glucose can be observed. Ferrous solid whose upper layer contains lactose can be used to observe lactose fermentation and $H_2S$ production. The content of glucose is only 1/10 of that of lactose. If the bacteria only break down glucose, the production of acid would be less, and the medium's surface is oxidized due to contact with air, so the surface and underlying firstly become yellow, then the surface becomes red. If the bacteria break down disaccharide and produce acid and gas, the medium would show yellow, and produce bubbles. If bacteria produce $H_2S$, it reacts with $FeSO_4$, this will form a black FeS.

【Materials and Equipment】

(1) Patients' feces specimens.

(2) SS agar plates, semi-solid disaccharide iron medium, diagnostic serum of *Salmonella*

(3) 载玻片、酒精灯、接种环、温箱。

**【实验方法】**

(1) 粪便标本首先接种于增菌培养基（必要时）。

(2) SS 琼脂平板分离培养：将粪便标本分区划线接种于 SS 琼脂平板上，置于 37℃温箱中孵育 18~24h，取出平板观察细菌菌落生长情况。

(3) 半固体双糖含铁培养基接种：从 SS 琼脂平板上挑选致病性肠道杆菌的可疑菌落（较小、无色、半透明或黑色中心），接种在半固体双糖含铁培养基内，置于 37℃温箱中培养 18~24h 后，取出观察结果。

(4) 血清学鉴定——玻片凝集：根据细菌在半固体双糖含铁培养基内的生长情况，进一步用已知沙门菌或痢疾杆菌诊断血清进行血清学（玻片凝集）实验及其他生化反应实验，作出最后鉴定。

**【实验结果】**

几种常见致病性肠道杆菌在半固体双糖含铁培养基上的生长情况及血清学鉴定结果如下表所示（表 3）：

**表 3　常见致病性肠道杆菌在半固体双糖含铁培养基上的生长情况及血清学鉴定结果**

| 半固体双糖含铁培养基 | | 诊断血清 | | | | | 致病性肠道杆菌 |
|---|---|---|---|---|---|---|---|
| 上层乳糖 | 下层葡萄糖 | 伤寒杆菌 | 甲型副伤寒杆菌 | 乙型副伤寒杆菌 | 福氏痢疾杆菌 | 宋内痢疾杆菌 | |
| 不分解;产生 $H_2S$ 或不产生 | 分解;产酸,不产气,有动力 | + | − | − | − | − | 伤寒杆菌 |
| 不分解;不产生 $H_2S$ | 分解；产酸，产气,有动力 | − | + | − | − | − | 甲型副伤寒杆菌 |
| 不分解;产生 $H_2S$ | 分解；产酸，产气,有动力 | − | − | + | − | − | 乙型副伤寒杆菌 |
| 不分解;不产生 $H_2S$ | 分解;产酸,不产气,无动力 | − | − | − | + | − | 福氏痢疾杆菌 |
| 迟缓分解；不产生 $H_2S$ | 分解;产酸,不产气,无动力 | − | − | − | − | + | 宋内痢疾杆菌 |

and *Bacillus dysenteriae*, etc.

(3) Slides, alcohol lamp, inoculation loop, thermostat.

**【Methods】**

(1) Firstly inoculate feces specimens in enrichment medium (if necessary).

(2) Isolated culture on SS agar plate: Inoculate feces specimens on different partitions of SS agar plate, incubate in 37℃ thermostat for 18–24h, then observe the growth of bacteria colonies.

(3) Inoculation of bacteria in semi-solid disaccharide iron medium: Choose pathogenic *Enterobacteriaceae* colonies on SS agar plate (smaller, colorless, transparent or black center), inoculate in semi-solid disaccharide iron medium, culture in 37℃ thermostat for 18–24h, observe the result.

(4) Serological identification—slide agglutination: According to the growth of bacteria in semi-solid disaccharide iron medium, apply the known diagnostic serum of *Salmonella* or *Bacillus dysenteriae* to perform serological test or other biochemical tests, and make the final identification.

**【Results】**

The growth of several common pathogenic *Enterobacteriaceae* in semi-solid disaccharide iron medium and results of serological identification are shown in the following table (Table 3):

Table 3 The Growth of Several Common Pathogenic *Enterobacteriaceae* in Semi-solid Disaccharide Iron Medium and Results of Serological Identification

| semi-solid disaccharide iron medium | | diagnostic serum | | | | | pathogenic *Enterobacteriaceae* |
|---|---|---|---|---|---|---|---|
| lactose in upper layer | glucose in bottom layer | *Salmonella typhi* | *Salmonella paratyphi A* | *Salmonella paratyphi B* | *Shigella flexneri* | *Shigella sonnei* | |
| don't break down; produce $H_2S$, or no $H_2S$ | break down; produce acid, no gas, move | + | – | – | – | – | *Salmonella typhi* |
| don't break down; no $H_2S$ | break down; produce acid and gas, move | – | + | – | – | – | *Salmonella paratyphi A* |
| don't break down; produce $H_2S$ | break down; produce acid and gas, move | – | – | + | – | – | *Salmonella paratyphi B* |
| don't break down; no $H_2S$ | break down; produce acid, no gas, don't move | – | – | – | + | – | *Shigella flexneri* |
| break down slowly; no $H_2S$ | break down; produce acid, no gas, don't move | – | – | – | – | + | *Shigella sonnei* |

# 实验二十二　试管凝集反应

**【实验目的】**

熟悉试管凝集反应的基本原理、方法和结果判定。掌握倍比稀释的方法和血清凝集效价/滴度的定义。

**【实验原理】**

用已知的诊断抗原与一系列倍比稀释后的待测血清在试管内混合，经一定时间保温反应后，观察每管是否出现凝集及各管的凝集程度，来定量检测待测血清中有无相应抗体及抗体的效价。

**【实验器材】**

（1）伤寒患者血清（1:10 稀释）、伤寒杆菌 O 和 H 抗原、甲型副伤寒杆菌和乙型副伤寒杆菌 H 抗原、生理盐水。

（2）试管、试管架、滴管、吸管等。

**【实验方法】**

（1）取清洁小试管 32 支，排成四排，分别标记序号及“O”“H”“甲 H”及“乙 H”等字。

（2）用 lmL 吸管吸取生理盐水，每管加入 0.5mL。

（3）在每一排的第一支试管中都加入伤寒患者血清（1:10 稀释）0.5mL，混匀。

（4）倍比稀释每排血清，即从已加有血清的第一管中吸取 0.5mL，加入第二管，混匀后吸取 0.5mL 加入第三管，混匀后吸取 0.5mL 加入第四管……直至第七管，混匀后吸取 0.5mL 弃去，第八管不加血清作为实验对照管。此时，每排每管的容量均为 0.5mL，第一管至第七管的稀释倍数依次为 1:20，1:40，1:80，1:160，…，1:1 280。

（5）分别吸取伤寒杆菌 O 菌液 0.5mL，加入第一排的各试管中；分别吸取伤寒杆菌 H 菌液 0.5mL，加入第二排的各试管中；分别吸取甲型副伤寒杆菌 H 抗原 0.5mL，加入

# XXII. Tube Agglutination

**【Aim】**

Get familiar with the basic principle, methods and results of tube agglutination. Grasp the dilution method and the definition of serum agglutination titer.

**【Principle】**

A known diagnostic antigen mixes with a series of diluted testing serum in tubes , and after a certain period of time, observe whether every tube shows agglutination and its aggregation degree, to detect whether testing serum contains the corresponding antibody and the titer of antibody.

**【Materials and Equipment】**

(1) Typhoid patients' serum (1:10 dilution) , *Salmonella typhi* containing O and H antigens, *Salmonella paratyphi A* and *Salmonella paratyphi B* suspension containing H antigens, and normal saline.

(2) Tube, test tube rack, dropper, straw, etc.

**【Methods】**

(1) Arrange 32 clean tubes in four rows, label them and tag"O" "H" "AH" and "BH" on them, respectively.

(2) Add 0.5mL normal saline per tube.

(3) Add 0.5mL typhoid patients' serum (1:10 dilution) in the first tube of each row, mix them.

(4) Dilute serums of each row: add 0.5mL serum to the second tube from the first tube, then mix it, take 0.5mL mixture from the second tube to the third tube, mix it, then take 0.5mL mixture from the third tube to the fourth tube, repeat this process. Finally, discard 0.5mL mixture from the seventh tube, and the eighth tube without serum as a control. The volume of each tube is 0.5mL, and the dilution ratio from the first to the seventh tube is 1:20, 1:40, 1:80, 1:160, ⋯, 1:1, 280, respectively.

(5) Add 0.5mL *Salmonella typhi* suspension containing O antigen to each test tube of the first row; add 0.5mL *Salmonella typhi* suspension containing H antigen in each tube of the second row; add 0.5mL *Salmonella paratyphi A* suspension containing H antigen in each tube of the third row; and add 0.5mL *Salmonella paratyphi B* suspension containing H antigen to each tube of the fourth row. At this point, dilution ratio of tubes of each row are

第三排的各试管中；分别吸取乙型副伤寒杆菌 H 抗原 0.5mL，加入第四排的各试管中。此时，每排各试管的血清稀释度依次为 1:40，1:80，…，1:2 560。

(6) 将各试管振荡混匀，连同试管架置于 56℃水浴箱中水浴 2~4h。

(7) 小心取出试管架，手持试管（切记不要混匀）对光观察试管内液体混浊度与管底凝集物的性状，以判断结果。

**【实验结果】**

第八管对照管为阴性反应，以“++”阳性反应的最高稀释倍数为血清抗体的效价（表 4）。

**表 4　试管内液体混浊度与管底凝集物的性状**

| 阳性反应 | 上层液体混浊度 | 管底凝集物 |
|---|---|---|
| ++++ | 完全澄清 | 凝集块很多，完全沉于管底 |
| +++ | 微呈混浊 | 凝集块很明显，大部分沉于管底 |
| ++ | 稍混浊 | 凝集块较多，中等量沉于管底 |
| + | 较混浊 | 凝集块较少，少部分沉于管底 |
| – | 混浊 | 没有凝集块，细菌沉于管底呈小圆点状 |

**【注意事项】**

(1) 要严格掌握时间，延长或缩短时间都会造成结果不准。

(2) 加样器吸取不同液体时，要及时更换吸头。

1:40, 1:80, ···, 1:2,560.

(6) Mix all tubes and incubate at 56℃ water bath for 2–4h in the test tube rack.

(7) Carefully take out of the tube rack, hold the tube with hand (do not mix) and observe the turbidity of the liquid and characteristics of the agglutinator in each test tube, to judge the result.

**【Results】**

The eighth tube is negative, and the highest dilution ratio showing a "+ +" positive reaction is determined as the antibody titer (Table 4).

Table 4 Liquid Turbidity and Agglutination Characteristics in Test Tubes

| positive reaction | the turbidity of upper liquid | agglutinator |
|---|---|---|
| ++++ | brilliantly clear | many agglutinator, entirely sink at the bottom of the tube |
| +++ | a little cloudy | agglutinator is so obvious that most of it is at the bottom of the tube |
| ++ | slightly cloudy | agglutinator is more, medium amount of it is at the bottom of the tube |
| + | more cloudy | agglutinator is little, a small amount of it is at the bottom of the tube |
| – | cloudy | no agglutinator, bacteria sink at the bottom of the tube which looks like a small round dot |

**【Attentions】**

(1) Strictly control testing time, if time is extended or shortened, the results would be inaccurate.

(2) When adding different liquid by a pipette, the tip must be replaced.

# 实验二十三 厌氧芽胞梭菌

## 一、厌氧培养法

【实验目的】

掌握疱肉培养基厌氧培养法和碱性焦性没食子酸厌氧培养法。

### (一) 疱肉培养基厌氧培养法

【实验原理】

培养基中的肉渣含有不饱和脂肪酸和谷胱甘肽，具有还原性，能吸收培养基中的氧，使氧化还原电势下降。又因以凡士林封闭培养基液面，故可防止空气中的游离氧进入培养基内，形成良好的厌氧条件，适于培养厌氧菌。

【实验器材】

(1) 破伤风梭菌、产气荚膜梭菌疱肉培养物。

(2) 疱肉培养基。

(3) 接种环、酒精灯、温箱。

【实验方法】

(1) 用接种环分别挑取破伤风梭菌、产气荚膜梭菌疱肉培养物两环，接种于疱肉培养基中（接种方法同前）。

(2) 置于37℃温箱中培养24~28h，观察细菌生长情况，注意培养基的混浊度，肉渣有无变化，有无气体产生。

【实验结果】

(1) 破伤风梭菌：生长良好，培养液变混浊，肉渣部分消化，微变黑，有少量气体。

(2) 产气荚膜梭菌：生长迅速，培养液变混浊，肉渣呈粉红色，不被消化，产生大量气体，将培养基表面的凡士林冲向试管口。

# XXIII. *Anaerobic Clostridium*

## i . Anaerobic Culture

**【Aim】**

To master cooked meat medium anaerobic culture method and alkaline pyrogallol anaerobic culture method.

### 1. Cooked Meat Medium Anaerobic Culture Method

**【Principle】**

The meat residue in the culture medium contains unsaturated fatty acids and glutathione, which have the reduction ability, and can absorb oxygen in the medium, so that the redox potential can be reduced. Because vaseline is layed on top of the culture, free oxygen in the air can be prevented from getting into the culture, forming good anaerobic conditions, suitable for culture of anaerobic bacteria.

**【Materials and Equipment】**

(1) Cooked meat cultures of *Clostridium tetani, Clostridium perfringens.*

(2) Cooked meat medium.

(3) Inoculation loop, alcohol lamp, thermostat.

**【Methods】**

(1) Take two loops of cooked meat cultures of *Clostridium tetani* and *Clostridium perfringens*, respectively, and inoculate them into cooked meat medium.

(2) Culture in a 37℃ thermostat for 24–28h, and observe the growth of bacteria. The followings, such as turbidity of the medium, whether the meat residue is changed, and whether gas is produced, shall be checked.

**【Results】**

(1) *Clostridium tetani*: good growth, medium becomes cloudy, meat residue is partially digested, and turn into blackish, with a small amount of gas produced.

(2) *Clostridium perfringens*: rapid growth, medium becomes cloudy, meat residue is not digested and in pink, large amount of gas is produced and push the vaseline cover on medium surface toward tube mouth.

### （二）碱性焦性没食子酸厌氧培养法

【实验原理】

焦性没食子酸是还原剂，在碱性溶液中能迅速吸收氧气，生成深棕色的焦性没食子橙，在培养皿内形成厌氧环境。

【实验器材】

(1) 破伤风梭菌、产气荚膜梭菌疱肉培养物。

(2) 血琼脂平板培养基。

(3) 无菌纱布块、脱脂棉、焦性没食子酸、10%NaOH 溶液、石蜡等。

(4) 平皿、接种环、温箱、酒精灯等。

【实验方法】

(1) 将细菌划线接种于琼脂平板上。

(2) 取方形玻璃一块，中央置脱脂棉一片，放 1 克焦性没食子酸于脱脂棉上，然后覆盖一小块无菌纱布，再向纱布上滴加 10%NaOH 溶液约 1mL。

(3) 立即将种有细菌的平板反盖于方形玻璃上，并把平板四周迅速用融化的石蜡密封。

(4) 置于 37℃温箱中培养 24~28h，取出，观察菌落特点及有无溶血现象等。

【实验结果】

(1) 破伤风梭菌：在血琼脂平板上呈扩散生长，菌落扁平、灰白色、边缘不齐、周边疏松似“羽毛状”，有狭窄溶血环，不易见到单个菌落。

(2) 产气荚膜梭菌：在血琼脂平板上形成圆形、凸起、表面光滑、边缘整齐的菌落。多数菌株有双层溶血环，内环呈 β-溶血，外环为 α-溶血。

## 二、破伤风梭菌、产气荚膜梭菌与肉毒梭菌的形态及染色性

【实验器材】

(1) 破伤风梭菌、产气荚膜梭菌和肉毒梭菌革兰染色标本片。

(2) 普通光学显微镜、镜油、擦镜纸。

【实验方法】

分别取三种细菌的革兰染色标本片，置于显微镜下观察其形态与染色性。

【实验结果】

(1) 破伤风梭菌为细长杆菌，芽胞为正圆形，直径比菌体宽度大，位于菌体顶端，使细菌呈“鼓槌状”，革兰染色阳性。

### 2. Alkaline Pyrogallol Anaerobic Culture Method

**【Principle】**

Pyrogallol is a reducing reagent, which can quickly absorb oxygen in alkaline solution and generate dark brown pyrobitumen gallic orange, making an anaerobic environment in the plate.

**【Materials and Equipment】**

(1) Cooked meat cultures of *Clostridium tetani, Clostridium perfringens.*

(2) Blood agar plate medium.

(3) Sterile gauze, absorbent cotton, pyrogallol, 10% NaOH solution, paraffin, etc.

(4) Plate, inoculation loop, thermostat, alcohol lamp, etc.

**【Methods】**

(1) The bacteria are streaked onto agar plate.

(2) Put a piece of cotton at central position of a piece of square glass, and add one gram of pyrogallol on cotton, then cover with a small piece of sterile gauze, again drop about 1mL of 10% NaOH solution on gauze.

(3) Immediately invert the streaked plate over the square glass and seal with melted paraffin.

(4) Incubate at 37℃ thermostat for 24–28h, and observe the colony characteristics and the presence of hemolysis phenomena.

**【Results】**

(1) *Clostridium tetani*: show diffusion growth on blood agar plate. Colonies are flat, gray. Edge is uneven, loose like "feather", with narrow hemolysis ring. It's not easy to see a single colony.

(2) *Clostridium perfringens*: form round, raised, smooth, neat edged colonies on blood agar plate. Most strains have double hemolysis rings, the inner ring is β-hemolysis, the outer ring is α-hemolysis.

## ii. Morphology and Staining Characteristics of *Clostridium Tetani, Clostridium Perfringens* and *Clostridium Botulinum*

**【Materials and Equipment】**

(1) Gram-stained smears of *Clostridium tetani, Clostridium perfringens* and *Clostridium botulinum.*

(2) Ordinary optical microscope, immersion oil, lens paper.

**【Methods】**

Take the Gram-stained smears of three kinds of bacteria, and observe their morphology and staining characteristics under the microscope.

**【Results】**

(1) *Clostridium tetani* is slender Gram-positive bacillus. The spores are circular, with larger diameter than cell width, located at the end of the cell, so that the bacterium is "drumstick-like".

(2) 产气荚膜梭菌为粗大杆菌，单独存在或成双排列，菌体周围有明显荚膜（机体内标本），革兰染色呈阳性。

(3) 肉毒梭菌菌体粗大，芽胞椭圆形，直径大于菌体宽度，位于次极端，使细菌呈典型的“网球拍形”，革兰染色呈阳性。

(2) *Clostridium perfringens* is Gram-positive thick bacillus, arranged alone or in pairs. Obvious capsule can be observed around the bacterial body in tissue specimens.

(3) *Clostridium botulinum* is thick, Gram-positive bacterium. The spores are oval, with diameter greater than the cell width, located at sub-terminal end of cell, so the bacterium looks like typical "tennis racket".

# 实验二十四　分枝杆菌

## 一、结核分枝杆菌的培养特征

【实验目的】

掌握结核分枝杆菌的培养特征。

【实验原理】

结核分枝杆菌是引起人和动物患结核病的病原菌，为抗酸染色阳性。它是专性需氧菌，人工培养时最适宜的pH值为6.5~6.8，营养要求较特殊，必须在含有血清、卵黄、马铃薯、甘油以及某些无机盐类的罗氏培养基上才能生长，生长非常缓慢，3~4周才能形成肉眼可见的菌落。

【实验器材】

(1) 结核分枝杆菌改良罗氏培养基培养物。

(2) 结核分枝杆菌苏通液体培养基培养物。

【实验方法】

(1) 取结核分枝杆菌改良罗氏培养基培养物，观察其生长情况，注意菌落特点。

(2) 取结核分枝杆菌苏通液体培养基培养物，观察其生长情况，注意液体表面生长特点。

【实验结果】

结核分枝杆菌在固体培养基上菌落干燥、坚硬，呈颗粒状、乳白色或米黄色，不透明，表面呈皱纹状，形似花菜心；在液体培养基内呈表面生长，形成皱襞状菌膜。

## 二、肺结核患者痰标本的直接涂片检查

【实验目的】

掌握肺结核患者痰标本直接涂片检查的原理、结果判断。

【实验原理】

分枝杆菌属的细菌，如结核分枝杆菌和麻风分枝杆菌，细胞壁中含有大量类脂（如

# XXIV. *Mycobacterium*

## i. The Culture Characteristics of *Mycobacterium Tuberculosis*

【Aim】

To master the culture characteristics of *Mycobacterium tuberculosis*.

【Principle】

*Mycobacterium tuberculosis* is the causative pathogen for human and animal tuberculosis. It's positive in acid fast stain, and obligate aerobes. The most suitable pH is at about 6.5–6.8, with special nutritional requirements. It must be cultivated in enriched medium containing serum, egg yolk, potato, glycerol and some inorganic salts, and grow very slowly, taking 3–4 weeks to form visible colonies.

【Materials and Equipment】

(1) Culture of *Mycobacterium tuberculosis* on improved Lowenstein-Jensen medium.

(2) Culture of *Mycobacterium tuberculosis* in Sauton liquid medium.

【Methods】

(1) Observe the growth and characteristics of the colony on improved Lowenstein-Jensen culture medium.

(2) Observe the growth and characteristics of the colony on surface of Sauton liquid medium.

【Results】

The colonies of *Mycobacterium tuberculosis* on solid culture medium are dry, rough, granular, milky white or beige colored, opaque, corrugated surface, like the flower of Chinese flowering cabbage. In the liquid culture medium, it grows on the surface to form pellicle.

## ii. Direct Smear Examination of Sputum Samples of Pulmonary Tuberculosis Patients

【Aim】

To master the principle and the judgment of results of the direct smear examination of sputum samples of pulmonary tuberculosis patients.

【Principle】

The cytoderm of *Mycobacterium*, such as *Mycobacterium tuberculosis* and *Mycobacterium leprae*, contains a lot of lipid, and it is not easy to be stained by aniline dyes. After being

分枝菌酸），对苯胺染料一般不易着色。若加温或延长染色时间或提高染液浓度使其着色后，再用3%盐酸乙醇溶液处理也不易脱色。经此法染色后，结核杆菌及其他分枝杆菌呈红色，其他非抗酸菌和细胞杂质等均呈蓝色。抗酸染色法是特异性地针对分枝杆菌属细菌的鉴别染色法。抗酸染色阳性的细菌称为抗酸杆菌（acid-fast bacilli）。

**【实验器材】**

(1) 肺结核患者痰标本。

(2) 抗酸染色一液、抗酸染色二液、抗酸染色三液。

(3) 载玻片、酒精灯、接种环、普通光学显微镜、镜油等。

**【实验方法】**

(1) 用接种环挑取痰液中脓样黄绿色部分或血丝部分涂片（涂片略厚为宜），自然干燥后通过火焰固定。

(2) 用抗酸染色法染色。

(3) 吸干后，用油镜检查，注意细菌的形态、排列及染色性。

stained with heating, or prolonged dyeing time or increasing concentration of dye, 3% hydrochloric acid ethanol solution is not easy to destain them. After using aniline dyes, *Mycobacterium tuberculosis* and other *Mycobacterium* are red, the other non-acid-fast bacteria and cell impurities are blue. Acid-fast staining method is designated for the identification of *Mycobacterium*. The bacteria which are acid-fast staining positive, are known as acid-fast bacilli.

**【Materials and Equipment】**

(1) Sputum samples of pulmonary tuberculosis patients.

(2) Acid-fast staining solution 1, acid-fast staining solution 2, acid-fast staining solution 3.

(3) Slides, alcohol lamp, inoculation loop, ordinary optical microscope, immersion oil.

**【Methods】**

(1) With inoculation loop, pick yellow-green pus-like part or blood containing part of sputum samples to make a thick smear, fix with flame after air dry.

(2) Stain with acid-fast staining.

(3) After dryness, observe with oil immersion lens, pay attention to bacterial structure, arrangement and dyeing property.

# 实验二十五 螺旋体形态（示教）

**【实验目的】**

掌握钩端螺旋体、梅毒螺旋体镀银染色的特点。

**【实验原理】**

病原性螺旋体形态纤细，折光性强，未经染色时不易查见，用革兰染色法染色时不易着色。常用冯泰纳（Fontana）镀银染色法及暗视野检查法。

**【实验器材】**

(1) 钩端螺旋体涂片，镀银染色标本片。

(2) 梅毒螺旋体涂片，镀银染色标本片。

(3) 普通光学显微镜、镜油、擦镜纸。

**【实验方法】**

取上述两种螺旋体染色标本片，置显微镜下观察，注意其形态、螺旋特点及染色性。

**【实验结果】**

(1) 钩端螺旋体呈棕褐色，螺旋盘绕紧密且规则，但分不清楚，一端或两端弯曲如钩状，常使菌体屈曲呈 C、S 等字形。

(2) 梅毒螺旋体呈棕色，两端尖直，有 8~14 个呈锐角弯曲而规则的螺旋。

# XXV. The Morphology of Spirochetes (Demo)

**【Aim】**

To master the characteristics of *Leptospira* and *Treponema pallidum* with silver staining.

**【Principle】**

Pathogenic spirochetes are morphologically slender and show strong refraction, but they are not easy to be found without staining. Gram staining method isn't effective. Fontana silver staining method or dark field examination method is often used.

**【Materials and Equipment】**

(1) *Leptospira* smears, specimens of silver staining.

(2) *Treponema pallidum* smears, specimens of silver staining.

(3) Ordinary optical microscope, immersion oil, lens paper.

**【Methods】**

Put the above two spirochetes' stained specimens under the microscope to observe the morphology, spiral characteristics and staining property.

**【Results】**

(1) *Leptospira* is brown in color. Its spirals are fine, tight and regular, and always bent like a hook at one end or both ends, presenting C or S-shaped.

(2) *Treponema pallidum*, is brown in color and straight at both ends. It has 8 to 14 bending and regular spirals in acute angle.

# 实验二十六 真菌基本形态及菌落特点

真菌（fungi）是真核细胞型微生物，可分为单细胞真菌和多细胞真菌两大类，单细胞真菌的结构较为简单，如新型隐球菌，是由母细胞发芽而繁殖；大多数真菌为多细胞，由菌丝和孢子两部分组成，由于菌种的不同，可出现不同形式的菌丝和孢子。由于真菌有特殊的形态和结构，一般根据其形态结构及培养特性即可对真菌进行分类鉴定。

**【实验目的】**

通过观察示教片，熟悉单细胞真菌和多细胞真菌的形态特点和培养特点。

**【实验原理】**

真菌分为单细胞和多细胞两种类型。前者细胞呈圆形或椭圆形，结构较为简单，如新型隐球菌、白色念珠菌等；大多数真菌为后者，多呈丝状，基本结构分为菌丝和孢子。真菌的菌落也与一般细菌不同，掌握真菌的形态结构和菌落特点对菌种分类鉴定有重要意义。

**【实验器材】**

（1）新型隐球菌墨汁负染标本。

（2）白色念珠菌涂片标本。

（3）须癣毛菌和石膏样小孢子菌涂片标本。

（4）新型隐球菌沙保斜面培养物。

（5）白色念珠菌沙保斜面培养物。

（6）絮状表皮癣菌沙保斜面培养物。

（7）普通光学显微镜、镜油、擦镜纸。

**【实验方法】**

（1）取新型隐球菌墨汁负染标本、白色念珠菌涂片标本，置于显微镜下观察，注意其形态特点。

（2）分别观察须癣毛菌及石膏样小孢子菌涂片标本，新型隐球菌、白色念珠菌及絮

# XXVI. Basic Morphology and Colony Characteristics of Fungi

Fungi are eukaryotic organisms which can be divided into unicellular fungi and multicellular fungi. The structure of unicellular fungi is relatively simple, such as *Cryptococcus neoformans*, which are sprouting from the mother cells. Most of the multicellular fungi are consisted of two parts: hyphae and spores. Due to the different species, there may be different forms of hyphae and spores. Usually fungi have special forms and structures, and they can be classified by morphological structures and culture characteristics.

**【Aim】**

Get familiar with the morphological and culture characteristics of unicellular fungi and multicellular fungi.

**【Principle】**

Fungi include unicellular fungi and multicellular fungi. The former cells are round or oval, and the structure is relatively simple, such as *Cryptococcus neoformans, Candida albicans*. Most of the fungi are the latter, with the basic structure of hyphae and spores. Fungal colonies are also different from those of most bacteria, so it is important to master fungal morphology and colony characteristics for the species identification.

**【Materials and Equipment】**

(1) Ink negative staining specimens of *Cryptococcus neoformans*.

(2) *Candida albicans* smear.

(3) Smears of *Trichophyton mentagrophytes* and *Microsporum gypseum*.

(4) Sabouraud slant culture of *Cryptococcus neoformans*.

(5) Sabouraud slant culture of *Candida albicans*.

(6) Sabouraud slant culture of *Epidermophyton floccosum*.

(7) Ordinary optical microscope, immersion oil, lens paper.

**【Methods】**

(1) Observe the specimens of ink negative staining *Cryptococcus neoformans* and *Candida albicans* smear under the microscope, pay attention to their morphological characteristics.

(2) Take the smears of *Trichophyton mentagrophytes*, *Microsporum gypseum*, the slant cultures of *Cryptococcus neoformans*, *Candida albicans* and *Epidermophyton floccosum*, observe their colony features.

状表皮癣菌沙保斜面培养物，注意其菌落特点。

【实验结果】

1. 形态特点

新型隐球菌菌体为球形，壁厚，大小不等，菌体周围有宽厚、透明的大荚膜；白色念珠菌菌体呈卵圆形，产生分枝的假菌丝，有厚膜孢子和芽生孢子；须癣毛菌可见小分生孢子群集于分枝菌丝末端，呈葡萄状，亦有圆形小分生孢子位于菌丝的侧旁；石膏样小孢子菌可见梭形具有横隔的大分生孢子。

2. 菌落特点

新型隐球菌菌落属酵母型菌落，圆形、较大、白色、边缘整齐、表面湿润光滑，与一般细菌菌落相似。

白色念珠菌菌落属类酵母样菌落，圆形、较大、白色，菌落底层有假菌丝长入培养基内。

絮状表皮癣菌菌落属于丝状菌落，表面有不规则隆起和浅沟，并有白色棉絮样气中菌丝，菌落的基底部呈茶褐色。

**【Results】**

## 1. Morphological characteristics

*Cryptococcus neoformans* are different-sized spherical cells with thick cell wall, and surrounded with thick, transparent large capsule. *Candida albicans* is oval, being able to produce branching pseudohyphae, chlamydospore and blastospore. *Trichophyton mentagrophytes* observed grape-like small clusters of spores on the end of branching hyphae, and there are spherical microconidiums located next to the side of mycelium. Macroconidiums with diaphragm can be seen in *Microsporum gypseum.*

## 2. Colony features

Colonies of *Cryptococcus neoformans* belong to yeast-type colony, they are similar to the bacterial colonies but with features of round, large, white, neat edges, smooth and moist surface.

Colonies of *Candida albicans* belong to yeast-like colony which is round, large, white with pseudohyphae underlying long into the culture medium.

Colonies of *Epidermophyton floccosum* belong to the filamentous colonies with irregular surface ridges and shallow trench and a white cotton-like hyphae, and colonies are dark brown at the bottom of the base.

# 实验二十七 病毒的形态学特点

## 一、病毒 CPE 观察

【实验目的】

熟悉病毒致细胞病变形态特点，了解其意义。

【实验器材】

(1) 正常人胚肾细胞培养物。

(2) 腺病毒感染后人胚肾细胞培养物。

【实验方法】

光镜下观察两种细胞培养物。

【实验结果】

正常人胚肾细胞呈多角形，单层排列。受腺病毒感染的细胞肿大变圆，细胞聚集成葡萄状，并可见细胞脱落现象。

## 二、病毒包涵体观察

细胞受某些病毒感染后，常可在其细胞浆或核内见到一些嗜酸性或嗜碱性圆形或椭圆形斑块状结构，称为包涵体。病毒感染形成的包涵体，因在组织细胞内定位不同及其本身的酸碱亲嗜性不同而具有鉴别诊断价值。

【实验目的】

了解狂犬病毒内基（Negri）包涵体的形态特点。

【实验器材】

(1) 狂犬病患犬海马部位神经组织病理切片经苏木素伊红染色标本片。

(2) 普通光学显微镜、镜油、擦镜纸。

【实验方法】

取狂犬海马部位神经组织病理切片经苏木素伊红染色标本片，置显微镜下观察，

# XXVII. Morphological Characteristics of Viruses

## i. Observation of Viral CPE

【Aim】

Get familiar with the morphological characteristics of virus caused cytopathy, and understand its significance.

【Materials and Equipment】

(1) Cultures of normal human embryonic kidney cells.

(2) Cultures of human embryonic kidney cells which are infected by Adenovirus(ADV).

【Methods】

Both cell cultures are observed under microscope.

【Results】

Normal human embryonic kidney cells are polygonal, arranged in monolayer. Adenovirus infected cells turned into round shape and accumulate to form grape-like structure, and some cells are detaching.

## ii. Observation of Viral Inclusion Body

Some round or oval eosinophilic or basophilic structures (called inclusion bodies) are often seen in cytoplasm or nucleus in some virus-infected cells. The formation of inclusion bodies with different positioning within the cells and the different pH tropism have diagnostic value after viral infections.

【Aim】

To know the morphological characteristics of inclusion body (Negri body) of rabies virus .

【Materials and Equipment】

(1) Hematoxylin-eosin stained specimens of hippocampus nerve tissue biopsy of dogs suffering rabies.

(2) Ordinary optical microscope, immersion oil, lens paper.

【Methods】

In order to understand the morphology, location and staining characteristics of rabies virus inclusion body, hematoxylin-eosin stained specimens of hippocampus nerve tissue biopsy of dog suffering rabies are observed under the microscope.

注意包涵体形态、存在部位及染色特点。

**【实验结果】**

神经细胞染成蓝色，狂犬病毒内基包涵体位于神经细胞浆内，嗜酸性，呈圆形或椭圆形，一个或数个，呈红色。

**【Results】**

Nerve cells are stained into blue, and inclusion bodies of rabies virus, called Negri body, are eosinophilic and stained into red. They are in round or oval shape and one or more Negri bodies can be observed in cytoplasm.

# 实验二十八　病毒的培养方法

病毒与细菌不同，它完全缺乏细胞器等必要装置，不能单独进行物质代谢，必须在易感染的活细胞中寄生，由宿主细胞供给其合成的原料、能量与场所才能增殖。

常用于病毒培养的方法有：易感动物接种法、鸡胚培养法和组织（细胞）培养法。下面仅介绍后两种。

## 一、鸡胚培养法

鸡胚培养法为常用的病毒培养方法之一，鸡胚培养法常用于病毒和立克次体的培养，用于痘类病毒、粘病毒和疱疹病毒的分离、鉴定，制备抗原，生产疫苗以及研究病毒性质等方面。其优点是操作简便、受精鸡卵来源丰富，鸡胚本身带病毒的情况少见，特别是鸡胚感染粘病毒后，在它的羊水和尿囊液中有大量的游离病毒存在，对动物红细胞可产生血凝现象，因此为初步鉴定病毒提供了一个依据。其接种方法有尿囊腔接种、绒毛尿囊膜接种、卵黄囊接种以及羊膜腔接种。

(1) 选卵：通常采用来亨鸡卵，其卵壳薄而色白，易于观察胚胎的生活情况；如不能得到，一般家鸡卵亦可用。

(2) 孵育：孵育前的卵，先用清水以毛刷洗刷清洁，用干布拭干，放入孵箱内进行孵育。适宜的孵育温度是 38~39℃，相对湿度是 45%~60%，并使空气流通，每日翻动鸡卵 1~2 次。

(3) 检卵：孵后第四天，用检卵灯检视鸡胚发育情况，捡出未受精及死亡的鸡卵，以后逐日检查其发育情况。

**【实验目的】**

(1) 熟悉鸡胚尿囊腔接种的方法及用途。

(2) 了解鸡胚接种的操作过程及有关技术。

**【实验原理】**

鸡胚和实验动物一样，为正常发育中的机体，有神经血管的分布及脏器的结构。鸡

# XXVIII. Cultural Methods of Viruses

Different from bacteria, viruses lack the necessary organelles and cannot metabolize independently. Viruses must live in susceptible living host cells, use the materials, energy and place which supplied by the host cell to proliferate.

Common methods used in culturing viruses are: susceptible animal inoculation method, chick embryo culture method and tissue (cell) culture method. We introduce the latter two methods.

## i. Chick Embryo Culture Method

The chick embryo culture method is one of the commonly used methods for virus culture. It is commonly used in the cultivation of viruses and rickettsiae, and to isolate, identify, and produce antigens and vaccine for poxvirus, myxovirus, herpes virus and so on. The advantages are: due to rich sources of fertilized chicken eggs and rare cases of embryo itself with the virus, chick embryo culture method is simple, especially after infected by myxovirus, there are large amount of free virus in amniotic and allantoic fluid of chick embryo. These viruses can cause animal erythrocytes produce clotting phenomenon, thus providing a basis for the preliminary identification of the virus. There are four methods of inoculation: allantoic cavity inoculation, chorioallantoic membrane inoculation, yolk sac inoculation and amniotic inoculation.

(1) Egg election: Leghorn chicken eggs are used usually because of their thin and white color egg shell which makes it easy to observe the living conditions of the embryo. If the leghorn chicken eggs cannot be gotten, the common chicken eggs can also be used.

(2) Hatching: before hatching, clean the eggs with water and wipe with a dry cloth firstly, then place them in the incubator. Suitable incubation temperature is 38–39℃, relative humidity is 45%–60%, and keeping air circulation, turning chicken eggs 1–2 times a day.

(3) Inspection of eggs: the fourth day after hatching, the inspection lamp are used to check chick embryos. Give up unfertilized eggs and dead eggs. Then check them every day.

**【Aim】**

(1) Be familiar with the methods and purposes of chick embryo allantoic cavity inoculation.

(2) Understand the procedures and related techniques of chick embryo inoculation.

胚来源充足，操作简便，通常是无菌的，对接种的病毒不产生抗体。对某些呼吸道病毒如正粘病毒、副粘病毒、痘类病毒、疱疹病毒和某些脑炎病毒很敏感，可用来从患者材料中分离上述病毒。

**【实验方法】**

(1) 选用 9~11 日龄鸡胚（此时尿液多，便于接种），在检卵灯上画出天然气室及鸡胚位置，在胚胎面与气室交界之边缘上约 0.5cm 处避开血管作一标记，此即为注射点。

(2) 用碘酒消毒后，用磨蛋器磨一小槽，磨破卵壳，不损伤壳膜。于注射点刺一小孔，针头与蛋壳成 30°，以短斜面针头自孔刺入 0.5~1.0cm，注入流感病毒（减毒株）0.1~0.2mL，然后用透明胶带封口，用蜡笔作标记，如图 22 所示。

(3) 置于 35~37℃温箱中孵育，每日照检一次，观察鸡胚的生长情况，在 24h 内死亡者应弃去，孵育 48~72h 后即可收获。取出放入 4℃冰箱，气室端向上，直立过夜，将鸡胚冻死使血液凝固，这样可避免在收获时流出的血细胞同尿液中的病毒发生凝集，造成病毒滴度下降。

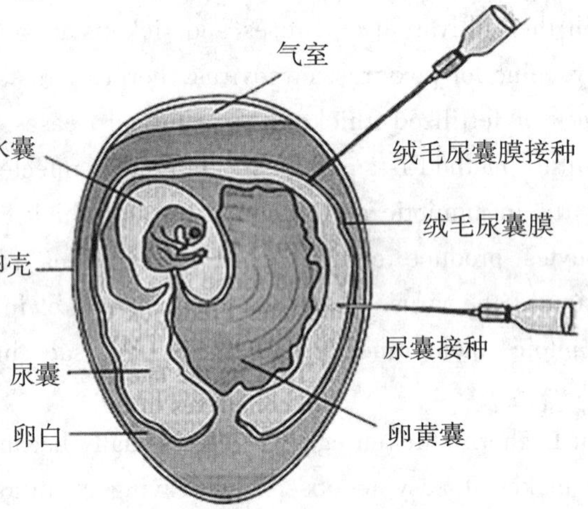


图 22 鸡胚培养法

**【实验结果】**

取出鸡胚，用碘酒消毒气室卵壳，用无菌剪刀击破气室端卵壳，用小镊子在无大血管处撕破卵膜，以无菌毛细管吸取尿囊液（一般可得 4~5mL），置于无菌试管中待做血凝实验、病毒鉴定及传代培养。同时应滴两滴尿囊液于无菌肉汤中做无菌实验。

## 二、细胞培养法

细胞培养法为病毒分离鉴定中最常用的方法。可根据细胞生长的方式分为单层细胞

**【Principle】**

Similar to experimental animals, chick embryos are individuals in normal development, possessing nerve, blood vessels and organs. Meanwhile, source of the chick embryo is sufficient, it is easy to operate and sterile, and no antibodies are produced against the inoculated virus. It is very sensitive to some respiratory viruses, such as orthomyxovirus, paramyxovirus, poxvirus, herpes virus and some encephalitis virus , and can be used to isolate the virus from the patient samples.

**【Methods】**

(1) 9 to 11-day-old chick embryos are selected (the urine is the most in this period which is convenient to inoculate) . The gas chamber and the position of chick embryo are drawn under inspection light. Mark the injection point which is about 0.5cm away from the junction edge of the embryo and the gas chamber.

(2) After disinfection, grind the egg shell and pierce a hole at the injection point, but do not damage shell membrane. During injection, the needle and eggshell is at a 30 degree angle, then from the hole piercing into 0.5 –1.0cm, injecting 0.1 –0.2mL influenza virus (attenuated strain), then sealed with transparent tape, and mark with crayon, it is shown in Figure 22.

(3) Place the eggs in 35 –37℃ thermostat. Inspect the living situation of the chick embryos once a day. Embryos die within 24h should be discarded and can be harvested after 48–72h. Put the eggs in 4℃ refrigerator and keep the air chamber up to stand overnight to kill the embryo and make blood clotting, which can avoid agglutination between blood cells and virus in the urine during collection. This agglutination will decrease the viral titers.

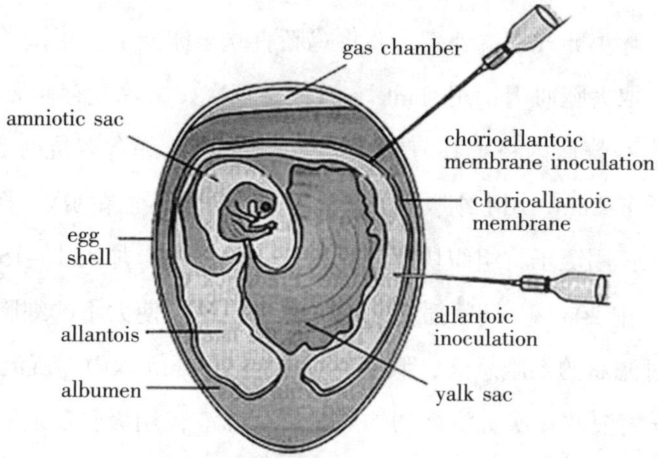


Figure 22 Chick Embryo Culture Method

**【Results】**

Remove the chick embryo, and scrub the gas chamber with iodine, then break the egg shell of gas chamber with sterile scissors, with a pair of tweezers tear egg membrane without

培养和悬浮细胞培养。从细胞的来源、染色体特征及传代次数等可分为：①原代细胞，来源于动物、鸡胚或引产人胚组织的细胞（如人胚肾细胞等），对多种病毒敏感性高，但来源困难；②二倍体细胞，指细胞在体外分裂 50~100 代后仍保持两倍染色体数目的单层细胞。③传代细胞系，由肿瘤细胞或两倍体细胞突变而来，能在体外持续传代，对病毒的敏感性稳定，因而被广泛应用。

鸡胚单层细胞培养

**【实验目的】**

(1) 熟悉细胞培养的方法及用途。

(2) 了解细胞培养的操作过程及有关技术。

**【实验原理】**

组织培养法是用离体活的器官、组织或细胞来培养病毒，是在体外培养单个细胞或单一性细胞群，并表现一定组织特性的培养方法。

**【实验器材】**

(1) 9~11 日龄鸡胚、流感病毒（减毒株）。

(2) Hank's 溶液、营养液、0.25%胰酶溶液。

(3) 无菌组织培养瓶、吸管、滴管、剪子、镊子、平皿、三角烧瓶等。

(4) $CO_2$ 培养箱、倒置显微镜等。

**【实验方法】**

(1) 用碘酒消毒鸡卵气室端外壳，并将鸡胚直立于卵架上。用镊子将小鸡取出，放在无菌培养皿内，取大腿肌肉，用 Hank's 溶液洗三次，去除残存血液。

(2) 用剪子在小烧瓶内将鸡胚剪成小块（1~2mm³），加含双抗的 Hank's 溶液（约 10mL）冲洗，静置 1~2min，用毛细吸管吸去液体，依同法再洗涤两次，将血液充分洗去。

(3) 胰酶消化：用镊子将组织块放入无菌三角烧瓶内，加入 10~15mL 0.25%胰酶溶液，置于 37℃水浴中 20min，期间摇动几次。由于胰酶可使大量的细胞游离，液体变混浊，经四层纱布过滤后的细胞悬液，低速离心（1 000r/min 以内）沉淀 5min，吸去上清液。再用 Hank's 溶液洗一次，沉淀物加入适量营养液，用吸管反复吹打细胞悬液，使细胞分散，再将细胞悬液通过不锈钢筛网，用白细胞计数的方法进行计数，使之成为每毫升含 50 万~80 万个细胞的细胞悬液。

(4) 在每个组织培养瓶中注入细胞悬液 1mL，盖好瓶塞，并将瓶略加摇动，横卧于有槽木架上，使细胞均匀平铺于瓶壁，置于 37℃温箱中孵育。一般 4h 后细胞即已附着

great vessel, transfer allantoic fluid(about 4–5mL) into sterile tubes for hemagglutination test, virus identification and culture. At the same time, add 2 drops of allantoic fluid in sterile broth for sterile test.

## ii. Cell Culture Method

Cell culture method is the most commonly used method in isolation and identification of viruses. Based on cell growth mode, this method can be divided into monolayer cell culture and suspension cell culture. Based on sources of cells, chromosomal properties and number of passages, etc. , it can be divided into: ①Primary cells, which are derived from animals, chick embryo or cells of induced human embryonic tissue (such as HEKC, etc. ). These kinds of cells are of high sensitivity to a variety of viruses, but they are difficult to get. ② Diploid cells. It is referred to monolayer cell which remain double chromosomes number after 50 to 100 generations' division in vitro. ③Passage cell lines. They are derived from cancer cells or mutant diploid cells. Because they can be continuous passaged in vitro and remain stable viral sensitivity, so they are widely used.

### Chick Embryo Cell Monolayer Culture

**【Aim】**

(1) Get familiar with the methods and purposes of cell culture.

(2) Understand the operation process and related techniques of cell culture.

**【Principle】**

Tissue culture is a method of culturing the virus in vitro with living organs, tissues or cells, and culturing a single cell or cell mass that can show certain organizational characteristics in vitro.

**【Materials and Equipment】**

(1) 9 to 11-day-old chick embryos, influenza virus(attenuated strain).

(2) Hank's solution, nutrient solution, 0.25% pancreatin solution.

(3) Sterile tissue culture flasks, pipette, dropper, scissors, tweezers, plates, narrow neck flask, etc.

(4) $CO_2$ incubator, inverted microscope.

**【Methods】**

(1) Disinfect the shell of the chicken egg's gas chamber with iodine, and put the eggs stand upright on holder. Remove the chick embryo with tweezers and place in a sterile Petri dish. Take the thigh muscle and wash three times with Hank's solution to remove residual blood.

(2) Cut chicken into small pieces(1–2mm$^3$) in a small flask, rinse with Hank's solution containing penniciline and streptomycin(about 10mL) . After stand for 1–2min, remove liquid with a capillary pipette. Repeat this step and wash three times till wash out all blood.

(3) Pancreatin digestion: The tissue pieces are clamped into a sterile narrow neck flask, then 10–15mL 0.25% pancreatin solution is added. Water bath at 37℃ for 20min and shake

于瓶壁，48h 已长成单层，此时即可弃去营养液，单层用 Hank’s 溶液洗两次，接种流感病毒，换以维持液。

**【实验结果】**

培养 48h 后长成单层，镜下可见瓶壁上有一层梭形活细胞，排列紧密，互相之间呈嵌合状，细胞外观透明，有一圆形核。受流感病毒感染的细胞肿大变圆，可见细胞脱落现象。

the flask several times. There are large amount of cells dissociated due to the effect of pancreatin. The liquid becomes turbid. Filter the cell suspension through four layers of gauze, and then centrifuge at low speed (1, 000r/min or less) for 5min to precipitate cells. Discard supernatant and wash cells with Hank's solution once. The precipitate is added an appropriate amount of the nutrient solution and scatter cells by pipette. Then the cell suspension is filtered through a stainless steel mesh. Adjust the concentration of cells to make sure there are 500–800 thousand cells per mL in this suspension.

(4) 1mL cell suspension is added into each tissue culture flask. Coverig the cork and slightly shake the flask. Then the flask is laid in the incubator and make sure the cells spread evenly on the inner side of the flask. The cells are incubated at 37℃. Generally, after 4h the cells has already attached to the wall of the flask, and will be monolayer after 48h. Discard the nutrient solution and wash the monolayer cells with Hank's solution twice, then inoculate influenza virus, and change to maintenance solution.

**【Results】**

After 48 hours of culture, cells become monolayer. Under the microscope, there is a layer on the sidewall of live fusiform cells which arrange closely to each other with fitted shapes. There is a circular core in this transparent cell. Influenza infected cells turned into round shape and some cells are detaching.

# 实验二十九　流感病毒的血凝与血凝抑制实验

## 一、血凝实验

**【实验目的】**

掌握血凝实验的原理及方法。

**【实验原理】**

由于各种病毒的性质不同及接种于鸡胚的部位不同，应采用不同的观察指标检测病毒的增殖情况。流感病毒颗粒表面有血凝素，具有使鸡、豚鼠血红细胞凝聚的能力。把一定浓度的鸡红细胞加到待检的鸡胚尿囊液或羊水中，如出现血细胞凝聚现象，即表示有病毒存在，这种实验称为血红细胞凝集实验，简称为血凝实验。

**【实验器材】**

(1) 已接种流感病毒的鸡胚。

(2) 0.5%鸡红细胞悬液、生理盐水、吸管、小试管、小镊子等。

**【实验方法】**

(1) 用镊子击破感染的鸡胚气室端卵壳，撕去壳膜，在无大血管处穿破绒毛尿囊膜，以无菌乳头吸管吸取尿囊液；如以羊膜腔接种法分离病毒时，则小心刺破羊膜，用吸管吸取羊水，放入无菌试管内，待检测。

(2) 取 10 支小试管在试管架上排成一行。

(3) 按表 5 所示加入各材料（均以 mL 为单位）。

(4) 摇匀，置室温 30~60min。

# XXIX. Hemagglutination and Hemagglutination Inhibition Test of Influenza Virus

## ⅰ. Hemagglutination Test

**【Aim】**

To master the principle and method of hemagglutination test.

**【Principle】**

Because the nature of different viruses and the site of inoculation in chick embryo, different index should be used to observe the proliferation of different viruses. Influenza virus has hemagglutinin on its surface, thus it has the ability to make red blood cells of chicken and guinea pig aggregate. Chicken red blood cell at certain concentration are added to the allantoic fluid or amniotic fluid. If blood cell aggregation occurs, it means the presence of virus, and this test is called red blood cell agglutination test, referred to as the hemagglutination test.

**【Materials and Equipment】**

(1) Chick embryo which are inoculated with influenza virus.

(2) 0.5% chicken red blood cell suspension, normal saline, straws, small tubes, tweezers, etc.

**【Methods】**

(1) Use tweezers to break up slightly the egg shell of the gas chamber of the infected chick embryo, remove the shell membrane, pierce into chorioallantoic membrane and avoid destroy large vessels. Suck up allantoic fluid with a sterile teat pipette and store in sterile test tube for detection. In the amniotic cavity inoculation method, the amniotic fluid is gathered and detected by piercing amniotic membrane.

(2) Take 10 small tubes and line up on the test tube rack.

(3) Add different reagents according to table 5 (unit: mL)

(4) Shake and place them at room temperature for 30–60min.

表 5 流感病毒血凝实验

| 试管 | 1 | 2 | 3 | 4 | 5 | 6 | 7 | 8 | 9 | 10 |
|---|---|---|---|---|---|---|---|---|---|---|
| 生理盐水 | 0.45 | 0.25 | 0.25 | 0.25 | 0.25 | 0.25 | 0.25 | 0.25 | 0.25 | 0.25 |
| 病毒液 | 0.05 | 0.25 | 0.25 | 0.25 | 0.25 | 0.25 | 0.25 | 0.25 | 0.25 | 弃 |
| 每管混匀后,吸出 0.25mL 移入下管中,第 9 管吸出 0.25mL 弃掉 | | | | | | | | | | |
| 稀释倍数 | 10 | 20 | 40 | 80 | 160 | 320 | 640 | 1 280 | 2 560 | 对照 |
| 0.5%鸡红细胞悬液 | 0.25 | 0.25 | 0.25 | 0.25 | 0.25 | 0.25 | 0.25 | 0.25 | 0.25 | 0.25 |
| 结果举例 | ++++ | ++++ | ++++ | +++ | ++ | ++ | + | – | – | – |

【实验结果】

(1) 首先观察对照管，红细胞应无凝集。

(2) 观察实验管，各管出现的红细胞凝集程度以“++++”“+++”“++”“+”“–”表示，判定标准如下：

++++：全部红细胞凝集，凝集的红细胞铺满管底，边缘不整齐。

+++：大部分红细胞凝集，在管底铺成薄膜状，但尚有少数红细胞不凝，在管底中心形成小红点。

++：约有半数红细胞凝集，在管底铺成薄膜，面积较小，不凝集的红细胞在管底中心聚成小圆点。

+：只有少数红细胞凝集，不凝集的红细胞在管底中心聚成小圆盘状，凝集的红细胞在此小圆盘周围。

–：不凝集，红细胞沉于管底，成一致密圆盘，边缘整齐。

凝集效价：能使红细胞呈++凝集的病毒的最高稀释度为凝集效价，表示含有一个单位血凝抗原。

## 二、血凝抑制实验

【实验目的】

掌握血凝抑制实验的原理及方法。

【实验原理】

流感病毒的血凝性，可被免疫血清中的特异性抗体所抑制，此实验称为血凝抑制实验，常用于流感病毒等粘病毒或副粘病毒的鉴定。

Table 5 Hemagglutination Test of Influenza Virus

| test tube | 1 | 2 | 3 | 4 | 5 | 6 | 7 | 8 | 9 | 10 |
|---|---|---|---|---|---|---|---|---|---|---|
| normal saline | 0.45 | 0.25 | 0.25 | 0.25 | 0.25 | 0.25 | 0.25 | 0.25 | 0.25 | 0.25 |
| virus solution | 0.05 | 0.25 | 0.25 | 0.25 | 0.25 | 0.25 | 0.25 | 0.25 | 0.25 | discard |
| after mixing, suck out 0.25mL into the next tube, discard 0.25mL in the ninth tube | | | | | | | | | | |
| dilution ratio | 10 | 20 | 40 | 80 | 160 | 320 | 640 | 1,280 | 2,560 | control |
| 0.5% chicken red blood cell suspension | 0.25 | 0.25 | 0.25 | 0.25 | 0.25 | 0.25 | 0.25 | 0.25 | 0.25 | 0.25 |
| examples of result | ++++ | ++++ | ++++ | +++ | ++ | ++ | + | – | – | – |

【Results】

(1) There is no red blood cell agglutination occur in the control tube.

(2) In experimental tubes, the degrees of agglutination are marked as ++++, +++, ++, + and –, which are judged according to the following standard:

++++: Hemagglutinating completely. The bottom of the tube is jaggedly covered with agglutinated red blood cells.

+++: Most hemagglutinating and form thin film at the bottom of the tube. But there are a small number of free red blood cells forming a red dot at the centre of the bottom.

++: About half hemagglutinating and form small thin film at the bottom of the tube. The free red blood cells gather together as a red dot.

+: Only a small number of red blood cells aggregating. Un-agglutinated red blood cells form a small round disk-shaped film in the center bottom of the tube, there are some agglutinated red blood cells around it.

–: No agglutination. Red blood cells sink to the bottom of the tube which form a dense disk with neat edge.

Agglutination titer is defined as the highest dilution of virus making ++ agglutination of red blood cells, indicating a unit containing hemagglutinin antigen.

## ii. Hemagglutination Inhibition Test

【Aim】

To master the principle and method of hemagglutination inhibition test.

【Principle】

Hemagglutinin of influenza virus can be inhibited by special antibody in the immune serum, the test about it is called hemagglutination inhibition test. This test is commonly used in the identification of myxovirus such as influenza virus or paramyxovirus.

【Materials and Equipment】

(1) Allantoic fluid of influenza virus infected chick embryo (4U / 0.25mL).

【实验器材】

（1）受流感病毒感染的鸡胚尿囊液（4U/0.25mL）。

（2）病人血清、0.5%鸡红细胞悬液、生理盐水、吸管、小试管等。

【实验方法】

（1）排列10支小试管于试管架上。

（2）按表6所示顺序等倍稀释诊断血清。（单位：mL）

（3）向各管加入流感病毒0.25mL。

（4）向各管加入0.5%鸡红细胞悬液各0.25mL。

（5）摇匀，置室温30~60min。

**表6　流感病毒血凝抑制实验**

| 试管 | 1 | 2 | 3 | 4 | 5 | 6 | 7 | 8 | 9 | 10 |
|---|---|---|---|---|---|---|---|---|---|---|
| 生理盐水 | 0.9 | 0.25 | 0.25 | 0.25 | 0.25 | 0.25 | 0.25 | 0.25 | 0.25 | 0.25 |
| 血清 | 0.1 | 0.25 | 0.25 | 0.25 | 0.25 | 0.25 | 0.25 | 0.25 | 弃 | 0.25(10×) |
| 每管混匀后，吸出0.25mL移入下管中，第8管吸出0.25mL弃掉 | | | | | | | | | | |
| 血清稀释倍数 | 10 | 20 | 40 | 80 | 160 | 320 | 640 | 1 280 | 病毒对照 | 血清对照 |
| 流感病毒 | 0.25 | 0.25 | 0.25 | 0.25 | 0.25 | 0.25 | 0.25 | 0.25 | 0.25 | – |
| 0.5%鸡红细胞悬液 | 0.25 | 0.25 | 0.25 | 0.25 | 0.25 | 0.25 | 0.25 | 0.25 | 0.25 | 0.25 |
| 结果举例 | – | – | – | – | – | ++ | ++++ | ++++ | ++++ | – |

【实验结果】

判定各管血细胞凝集的情况，方法与流感病毒血凝实验相同。鉴定病毒时，效价应与原免疫血清效价相等或相似。血凝抑制实验亦可用已知病毒检测血清抗体。测定病人血清抗体以进行血清学诊断，恢复期比初期抗体效价增高4倍以上才有诊断意义。

【思考题】

（1）血凝实验的原理是什么？

（2）流感病毒的鉴定方法有哪些？

(2) Patient's serum, 0.5% chicken red blood cell suspension, normal saline, straws, small tubes and so on.

**【Methods】**

(1) Arrange 10 small tubes on the test tube rack.

(2) Dilute the serum in series according to table 6 (unit: mL)

(3) Add 0.25mL influenza virus to each test tube.

(4) Then add 0.25mL 0.5% chicken red blood cell suspension to each test tube.

(5) Shake and place them at room temperature for 30–60min.

Table 6 Hemagglutination Inhibition Test of Influenza Virus

| test tube | 1 | 2 | 3 | 4 | 5 | 6 | 7 | 8 | 9 | 10 |
|---|---|---|---|---|---|---|---|---|---|---|
| normal saline | 0.9 | 0.25 | 0.25 | 0.25 | 0.25 | 0.25 | 0.25 | 0.25 | 0.25 | 0.25 |
| serum | 0.1 | 0.25 | 0.25 | 0.25 | 0.25 | 0.25 | 0.25 | 0.25 | discard | 0.25(10×) |
| after mixing, suck out 0.25mL into the next tube, discard 0.25mL in the eighth tube | | | | | | | | | | |
| dilution ratio | 10 | 20 | 40 | 80 | 160 | 320 | 640 | 1,280 | virus control | serum control |
| influenza virus | 0.25 | 0.25 | 0.25 | 0.25 | 0.25 | 0.25 | 0.25 | 0.25 | 0.25 | — |
| 0.5% chicken red blood cell suspension | 0.25 | 0.25 | 0.25 | 0.25 | 0.25 | 0.25 | 0.25 | 0.25 | 0.25 | 0.25 |
| examples of result | – | – | – | – | – | ++ | ++++ | ++++ | ++++ | – |

**【Results】**

To determine the hemagglutination in each tube by using the same method as the influenza virus hemagglutination test. In the identification of virus, the titer should be equal or similar to original immune serum. Hemagglutination inhibition test can also use a known virus antigen to measure serum antibodies for serological diagnosis. But only when recovery titer increased more than four times than the initial antibody titer, the diagnostic significance is meaningful.

**【Questions】**

(1) What is the principle of hemagglutination test?

(2) What are the influenza virus identification methods?

